II EMPLOYMENT

III COUNSELLING

Preface

The *How To Do It* series has proved very popular, both in its regular appearance in the *BMJ* and as a series of three volumes. Some chapters have stood the test of time, being as relevant now as they were up to 15 years ago, but most subjects have moved on. We therefore thought that we should ask the original authors to update their chapters. Where this was not possible we commissioned new authors. We have included articles that have been published in the *BMJ* since the last volume was published and added chapters on new topics as they presented themselves. New authors worked hard to preserve an existing style while adding something of themselves.

Considering the old and the new articles together points up some interesting changes in writing style since the late 1970s. No longer is it acceptable to refer to all doctors as "he" and use expressions such as "the ladies' programme" for conferences. It's not only political correctness but also reflects the larger number of women entering the profession – and reading these books. But more difficult to explain is the fact that the new contributions have become more serious, their authors keener to provide a comprehensive account.

The health service has itself changed. Recent reforms have altered procedures, structures, and people's jobs. Emphases have shifted, and some topics such as audit, have grown so much that covering it in a single chapter was impossible. Doctors now increasingly recognise the importance of management, and this is reflected in the revisions and new chapters.

In the previous editions the order of publication in the *BMJ* dictated the order the chapters appeared in the books. The new editions gave us the opportunity to group the chapters together with some sort of logic. The three volumes of the series now have individual themes. This first volume covers the broad categories of management, employment, and counselling. An enormous amount of helpful information is gathered here, not only for juniors who want to know how to write a curriculum vitae and perform well in interviews but also for senior doctors who need to improve their dictating technique or appoint a colleague. There is valuable advice for those who want to start in private practice, job share, or be a locum. The section on counselling outlines what death means in certain ethnic groups and gives guidelines on dealing with patients with cancer.

There are generous lashings of culture, particularly from Hugh Baron and Douglas Black, and light relief from others. Many will appreciate Jim Drife's tongue-in-cheek advice not to wear a bow tie or suede shoes to an interview; the late John Stallworthy's bitter experience of an appointed candidate not living up to his reference; and Anne Savage's suggestion that old *BMJ*s should be used for toilet paper when desperate – and abroad.

I would like to thank all of the contributors, old and new, for writing so well and so willingly. I would also like to acknowledge Helen Bodenham, our editorial assistant, who has revealed a detective's talent for tracking down authors, without which these books would be – well – smaller.

DEBORAH REECE
January 1995

I MANAGEMENT

1 Be a manager

Cyril Chantler

There is no right or wrong way to learn how to be a manager, and in this respect management is quite different from medicine or science. My qualification for being asked to write this chapter was that I had spent three years as chairman of the Guy's Hospital management board, with the title of Unit General Manager, but without any specific training. I had read a book while on a long journey before taking up my appointment,[1] which, in retrospect, was insufficient. Training is dealt with more fully below, but I will state now that the best book on management, which I read soon after taking up my appointment, is Sir John Harvey Jones's *Making It Happen*.[2] I recommend this to any clinician or academic because it emphasises the importance of leadership, with its characteristics of imagination, courage, and sensitivity. Management is not the same as command or administration, but it requires characteristics derived from both. I am mostly concerned with the contribution that clinicians can make to the success of the NHS.

Qualifications

Many doctors have management experience, though they commonly discount this and spend little time analysing it. Most will have been required to organise activities on behalf of others at school, at university, or in practice. They are also experienced at making difficult decisions with inadequate information. They learn to live

3

with the consequences while being prepared to accept that when they are wrong they must try again, driven by their responsibility for other people's lives and health. Sometimes they find it difficult to accept that management, like medicine, is an inexact science. At least as far as hospitals are concerned, management is as important as medicine because doctors can serve their patients only if the resources are available and the whole team is organised to work at maximum efficiency.

Clinicians are natural leaders in a hospital. They, more than any other group, make the decisions that most affect the activities of the whole organisation. Consultants are usually associated intimately with a single hospital over many years. They are well educated and intelligent (intelligence being a necessary criterion for entry to the profession), and undoubtedly develop stamina in the early years after qualification. A sense of humour, if not natural, is certainly a common defence against the tensions of the job. All of these characteristics are useful for a manager. Doctors and managers ought to be good listeners: active listening is essential for obtaining a clinical history from a patient, which enables the nature of a problem to be defined clearly in a relatively brief time. Doctors concerned with management are, surprisingly, not always as skilled as might be expected at counselling staff and making decisions that may affect employees profoundly. Sometimes a natural loyalty to people hampers decisions that are vital to the hospital. It is no use keeping people in jobs that are not necessary or in which their performance is poor; it is far better to help them by analysing their performance, providing motivation, retraining them, or occasionally allowing them to leave with proper entitlements.

By far the most important qualification for a good manager is the ability to establish and lead a team. No matter how talented any individual might be, this is rarely, if ever, an adequate substitute for the combined efforts of a team of people working together. Team leadership and team thinking skills can be acquired through training and coaching, and can be constantly improved. A most useful book that deals with this aspect of management is *The Professional Decision Thinker and the Art of Team Thinking Leadership*.[3] It emphasises the importance of bringing together a group of people concerned with a particular problem, making sure that they have the same understanding of the basis of the problem and work through possible solutions, encouraging everyone's ideas and testing them formally against alternatives before selecting the best solution.

Strategy and structure

It is always worth spending a great deal of time thinking and talking about the strategy of the organisation and making sure the structure is, or remains, correct. In 1984 Guy's Hospital was faced with a reduction in its budget of nearly 20% over eight years. The previous five years had been characterised by closures of beds, inadequate replacement of equipment, little expenditure on the infrastructure of the hospital, and falling morale, with increasing antagonism between different professional groups. Consultant staff, angered by their inability to provide care and by problems ranging from lengthening waiting lists to the frequent absence of outpatients' records, made formal representations at all levels of the health service, and many of us took advantage of the proximity of Guy's Hospital to Fleet Street and the media to appeal to the public for more money for the NHS, but with little success. One consultant, however, succeeded in securing a donation to sustain his service for a year, and another set up an appeal fund that has continued to provide over £250 000 yearly to support the children's unit.

The crisis encouraged a deep analysis of strategy and structure. The most important question to be answered was whether clinicians should be concerned with the management of hospitals. The important characteristic of the NHS is that it is cash limited, unlike the private sector. Clinicians need resources if they are to have clinical freedom. An authority that is cash limited will not transfer responsibility for management to a group that refuses to accept financial responsibility, nor will it readily accept or act on advice from a medical advisory committee whose members are not financially aware or accountable. After much debate the clinicians at Guy's Hospital reached an agreement whereby they would accept financial responsibility and accountability in return for management authority. Parenthetically, they also realised that if they could show that the hospital was efficient they would have a stronger voice in determining the allocation of resources at all levels in the NHS.

There are four principles that, in my opinion, govern the participation of clinicians in management.

Professional and management accountability are different

To a greater extent than in most organisations, hospital staff are drawn from members of several very different professions. Nurses, administrators, scientists, engineers, catering staff, accountants, personnel officers, and doctors all have their own professional organisations that determine training and set standards and to which they are accountable. Traditionally, hospitals have been administered by a trio of a doctor, a nurse, and an administrator, with help from other professional groups. The head of each professional group is concerned largely with the performance of his or her own department or function and has only a secondary concern for overall management, rather like the leader of a section in an orchestra with no director or conductor. General management has to be seen in the light of the many different professional groups that constitute the staff of a hospital.[4] No one person can hope to be competent in all areas. Mr Enoch Powell remarked that the Minister of Health has to accept advice from doctors without question whereas the Minister for Defence can contradict his generals.

Professional accountability must be protected, and certainly no interference by management in the care of a patient can or should be tolerated; the first responsibility of a doctor is to the patient. Management accountability is separate and different. The public has the right to know that the resources provided by taxation are being used efficiently and effectively and that everyone in the organisation is accountable managerially. In our structure staff continued to report professionally and to be accountable to their seniors; thus all nurses were accountable to the director of nursing. Managerially, the final responsibility was held by the chairman of the board, who was a doctor, and the directors of professional and administrative groups were accountable to him; he in turn was accountable to the district general manager and the district health authority.

Responsibility and authority must be commensurate

Large hospitals are too complex to be managed centrally. A number of different systems have been developed in order to encourage successful decentralisation. A number of recent publications deal with this issue.[5, 6] In 1985 we decentralised to 14 clinical directorates, each managed by a team of a nurse, a business manager, and a doctor, who headed it. Each directorate managed its own affairs as far as possible, and was responsible for the staff working within the directorate, including doctors, nurses, clerical staff, scientists, technicians, and record staff. Each directorate had its own ward or wards and organised its own admissions and outpatients. By the time the decentralisation process was complete in

1988, two-thirds of our staff reported within the directorates. Budgets were set yearly and there was a requirement to meet agreed targets of quantity and quality of patient care within the financial provision. However, responsibility that is decentralised must be accompanied by the transfer of sufficient authority to fulfil that responsibility. If power without responsibility is dangerous, then responsibility without authority is demoralising.

We were particularly concerned to keep lines of accountability as short as possible, in other words, to produce a "flat structure." Although our management board was large, with its 14 clinical directors, unit general manager, chief executive and functional directors such as nursing, finance, personnel, pharmacy, and works, it functioned effectively. In order to achieve this, a smaller management executive accountable to the board met weekly, and the board set up smaller groups to deal with specific problems and then to report back. This meant that the main board, which met monthly, never met for more than two hours at most and received papers that were well thought through and constructed before presentation. The advantage of having a large management board, bringing together both clinical and functional managers, was that strategic issues and operational issues could be dealt with in one forum, so that the traditional problem of the people at the top knowing what to do, but not knowing how to do it, and the people at the bottom knowing how to do things, but not knowing what to do was ameliorated. In 1985 a particular problem was the Salmon structure for nursing, with its long lines of accountability reducing the authority and managerial confidence of ward sisters. In the structure we developed clinical teams led by the ward sister and consultants working together, with their own budgets, reported directly to the clinical directorate concerned, thus taking management down to the level where it really matters, at the interface with patient care.

Part-time commitment

Clinical work requires practice, and clinicians in management should continue to maintain clinical duties for the benefit of their own professional future and satisfaction and because they can bring their unique perspective to management only if they do. Management and administration should not be confused. The clinician manager needs an administrator, who should be a colleague whose professional skills are valued. The relationship between the manager and the administrator can be viewed as similar to that between a minister and a permanent secretary.

Information and budgeting

Good management needs good information—for example, I was taught that the first action to take when a patient with diabetic ketoacidosis was admitted was to telephone the staff of the clinical chemistry laboratory and enlist their support. Good management also depends on doing the best you can with the information available. It is no use providing sophisticated information or clinical budgeting systems if there is no management structure that can use them. Our policy was to concentrate on getting the structure right. The new management board at Guy's Hospital, which started working in April 1985, inherited a yearly rate of overspending of about £5m. This was tackled by recognising that about 70% of expenditure was on staff and that the key pieces of information that we lacked were how many people we employed and how much they earned. Overspending is best approached by reducing costs and then allowing activity to adjust rather than the reverse. Having identified the role of each employee, we then reduced staffing by about 10% over six months while doing our best to protect clinical activity. One of the key tasks of the NHS is to regain the post-1948 enthusiasm for treating as many patients as possible to an acceptable standard rather than being led by the need to balance the books; balancing the books is essential but is not the purpose of the service. In the three years 1985–8 we reduced staffing by 17% and expenditure by 15% (£7m yearly) and by the end of the period had treated nearly 40 000 inpatients—more than ever before.

Accountancy in the NHS is traditionally functionally based; thus nursing staff, medical staff, clerical staff, maintenance and catering all had budgets even though they were mostly unmanageable by any one person. Reorganisation into multiprofessional management groups had to be followed by management accountancy so that each of these groups was provided with accurate information concerning income and expenditure. The change from a functional to a management accountancy system in the NHS is a major advance that has been achieved over the last few years. It does, however, take time to set up new systems, and the quality of the information improves only after an iterative process between the finance department and the clinically based manager. By April 1990 the clinical directorates and ward based clinical groups at Guy's were receiving monthly statements of expenditure set against budgets for staffing, sterile supplies, stores and consumables, drugs, repairs and maintenance, and consumables in pathology and radiology departments. The possibilities for improving efficiency should not be underestimated: a ward sister saved £5000 in nursing costs and £1300 in consumable costs on her ward each month. Later, the whole cost of pathology and radiology was further decentralised to the clinical groups, who then bought, at full cost, services from these various departments. Other possible developments in such a decentralised system would be to provide clinical directorates with the budgets for the use of intensive care, and operating theatres, and to develop an internal recharging system for the use of "borrowed beds".

Quality

As long as patients cannot receive the treatment they need when they need it, quantity must remain the most important aspect of quality in the NHS, but it should not be an excuse for poor quality. Improving quality can save money and improve clinical efficiency. Our decentralised outpatient appointment system, run by each firm's medical records and clinic clerk, led to better-spaced appointments, with reduced waiting times, less crowding, and therefore less pressure on the staff, no missing notes, and no fewer patients. Preadmission clinics for surgery with regular reviews of waiting lists can lead to fewer operations being cancelled. High occupancy of beds does not necessarily mean higher patient throughput, and we all know hospitals where patients are admitted early simply to "protect the bed". These are all aspects of management where only the doctor "can reach the parts that other managers fail to reach". Medical audit or clinical review should also be encouraged as a means to improve clinical efficiency as well as effectiveness.[7]

Time

Since a common argument used against concerning clinicians with management is lack of time, it is worth asking how much time is already spent in committee and whether this effort is productive. Using your own and others' time efficiently is an essential quality of management. Much can be achieved by a telephone conversation, by being rigorous about reading and keeping only essential material, by not having lots of minutes, by stating when a meeting will end as well as when it will start, and by delegation. It should be emphasised that time spent in determining operational policies is seldom wasted, and a well-organised clinical service will release time and resources for caring for patients. Management time for clinicians can often be created outside clinical sessions: surgeons like to meet before breakfast whereas physicians seem to prefer to meet at dinner; lunchtime is a good time to meet the non-clinical staff.

Listening

As a manager it is easy to become desk-bound and concerned with details to the extent that the main tasks pass you by. You should try to ensure that you keep definite periods free for visiting all parts of the hospital—"the best manure is the farmer's feet"—and you may find that visiting people in their own departments rather than meeting them in your office is useful and helps to put a problem into its proper context. You should be available to offer advice when problems occur; in the long run this can save a lot of time for yourself and the whole organisation. Dealing with mail efficiently and promptly is important, and generally I try to ensure that my desk is clear at the end of each day.

Decisions and leadership

A good manager has to be decisive, but not all decisions will be correct, and there is often no harm in admitting that you were wrong and trying again. A good decision will command support among all those who have to implement it, and, indeed, they should have helped to formulate it. Often a properly led discussion will produce an obvious decision; at other times competing priorities will preclude a consensus, but the decision, once made, will still be carried through as long as everyone is satisfied that it has been properly reached.

A clinical manager has an important leadership role. Leadership implies that there are those who are prepared to follow. The clinical directors and the chairman of the board at Guy's were appointed not elected, but it was clear that if they lost the support of their colleagues they would have little option other than to resign and be replaced. Checks on the possible abuse of authority are important, and the British system of all consultants being created equal is too valuable to discard.

Incentives and motivation

A defect of the NHS is the lack of incentive to good performance at all levels. Far too many people earn far too little and work far too ineffectively. We need the freedom to pay people according to performance and can look to do so by using the resources released by employing fewer people. Even under the present system a little imagination can be helpful, and the recent changes in the all-embracing and suffocating Whitley system are to be welcomed. A good manager will be looking for ways to increase motivation, and should not underestimate the devotion to patient care of all staff in the NHS. Most people who work in the service are proud of it and are underappreciated; showing that you, the manager, appreciate their efforts is vital.

Everyone in the organisation should understand their job, should know to whom they report, and should have their performance reviewed regularly to provide motivation, advice, and help. A formal staff development or appraisal system is useful. The flow of information up and down the organisation can be improved by a system of team briefing.[8] Social occasions are important, and an occasional chat over a drink can often be invaluable.

Nothing causes so much uncertainty or hostility in a hospital as a reorganisation of office, clinic, or ward space. None the less, it is vital that staff in management teams work near each other so that communication is facilitated. Key staff in the central management, such as the clinician manager, chief administrator, director of nursing, financial director, and personnel director, must have their offices near each other.

Training

I have already suggested that clinicians have more management experience than they might realise. They need to have a general appreciation of how the NHS works and the roles and skills of other professionals. Much can be learnt from informal discussions with finance staff, administrators, and personnel officers.

Since the clinical directorate system was introduced a number of useful publications have been produced.[9, 10, 11] The British Association of Medical Managers (BAMM, Bernes Hospital, Cheshire) brings together all doctors who are interested or involved in management, and anyone interested should be encouraged to join.

It runs a number of training days and courses as well as an annual conference and produces a quarterly journal. Other courses are run by bodies such as the King's Fund College, the Royal College of Physicians, the NHS Training Authority and business schools throughout the country. These courses can be useful not only because of what is taught, but also for the chance to meet others with similar responsibilities and to reflect on problems.

Some management awareness, if not specific training, is now being introduced into the undergraduate curriculum, and newly qualified doctors and junior staff should be encouraged to be involved at an early stage, through participating in clinical audit and resource management within a clinical directorate. More specific training is appropriate during higher professional training, and newly appointed consultants who are interested in participating in management should be encouraged. This interest in management does not need and should not be allowed to interfere with the main professional task of caring competently for one's patients.

Some clinicians, particularly as their career develops, may wish to develop a stronger interest in management and, indeed, become full-time or almost full-time managers. They can eventually become chief executives of trusts or purchasing authorities. More than one doctor has been or is a regional general manager and for such individuals more specific training in management is appropriate.

Conclusion

These continue to be critical times for the NHS. The gap between demands for the provision of care and the available funding continues to widen and increasingly more and more difficult choices have to be made. The proportion of national wealth spent on the NHS has risen sharply and is now 6.6% of gross domestic product, which correlates closely with the proportion spent by other developed countries, at least in relation to per capita income. Whatever further changes are devised in the management of the NHS to deal with these difficult pressures, no one can doubt the need for competent management of the available resources. It is therefore in the interests of patients as well as doctors that clinicians should participate in the management of their hospitals. A team approach that uses the skills of professionals and shares the responsibility for management with other colleagues by decentralisation offers the opportunity for clinicians to be managers without making it impossible for them to pursue clinical or academic practice. Obviously we need to argue for more money for the NHS and a greater share of the national revenue. We are more likely to obtain this if we can show clinical efficiency and maintain the support of the public by providing a more personal and convenient service. Management is too important to be left to others; doctors must play a part.

1 Drucker P F. *Management*. London: Pan Books, 1977.
2 Harvey-Jones J. *Making it happen*. London: Collins, 1988.
3 Heirs B. *The professional decision thinker and the art of team thinking leadership*. London: Grafton, 1989.
4 NHS Management Inquiry. *Report*. London: Department of Health and Social Security, 1983. (Griffiths report)
5 British Association of Medical Managers, British Medical Association, Institute of Health Service Management and the Royal College of Nursing. *Managing clinical services; a consensus statement of principles for effective clinical management*. London: Institute of Health Service Management (75 Portland Place, London W1N 4AN), 1993.
6 Wraith M, Casey A. *Implementing clinically based management; getting organisational change under way, a handbook for doctors, nurses and other hospital managers*. Droitwich: Wraith Casey Management Consultants (7 Vines Mews, Droitwich, Worcestershire WR9 8LE), 1992.
7 Hoffenberg R. *Clinical freedom*. London: Nuffield Provincial Hospital Trust, 1987:1–105.
8 Grummitt J. *Team briefing*, 2nd ed. London: Industrial Society, 1988.
9 Rea C, ed. *Managing clinical directorates*. Longman: 1993.
10 White T. *Management for clinicians*, London: Edward Arnold, 1993.
11 Burrows M, Dyson R, Jackson P, Saxton H, eds. *Management for hospital doctors*. Oxford: Butterworth-Heinemann, 1994.

2 Chair a committee

A G W Whitfield

One out of four telephone calls to a consultant finds him or her away at, or in, a meeting and incommunicado, and three out of four to an administrator meet the same fate (personal unpublished research). Some of the consultant's meetings are of an important clinical, scientific, or educational nature and some of the administrator's meetings are essential for the smooth working of a hospital, district, or region. However, committees have become an increasing preoccupation of the NHS and many of them serve little or no useful purpose. Democracy demands that everybody must be represented and in consequence committees grow larger and larger. The majority are held during time in which those attending are highly paid to do other work, considerable travel and subsistence expenses may be involved, and a secretariat is required. Moreover, the cost of producing and posting the agenda and other papers is considerable.

No one appears to have published any estimate of the proportion of the health service budget spent on committees; indeed like so many other NHS activities it would probably be impossible to do so with any degree of accuracy and even less feasible to assess their cost effectiveness. If the number of committees and the numbers serving on each committee could be reduced by one half, it would be unlikely to harm the service and it would release a vast amount of money and expert time for the real purpose of the health service—to care for the sick.

A request to be chairperson of a committee should not therefore always be regarded as a mark of the high esteem of one's colleagues and eagerly accepted as an appointment of distinction. It may well be that those requesting your services appreciate that the particular committee is a waste of time and that they have been rebuffed by six others already approached. Even committees that meet only quarterly demand considerable time and effort from the chairperson and secretary, and before accepting one should ask oneself three questions: Is the committee going to achieve anything? Have you the knowledge and ability to chair it? Could anyone else available do it better? Honest answers will certainly not leave you responsible for many committees.

Before you begin

An acceptance carries with it a heavy commitment if your appointment is to be a success. The time actually spent "in the chair" is small, but the necessary reading, discussion, consultation, persuasion, and cultivation of good relationships consume many hours. As a chairperson you are the most important member of the committee and you have to steer it and carry the other members with you. Your chief lieutenant, on whom you will be heavily dependent, is the committee secretary. If it is a university committee he or she will be a member of the registry, a graduate and someone with considerable personal qualities and experience. The quality of the secretariat provided for college committees is equally high and you will find yourself in safe and protective hands. Naturally, it is not always possible for the NHS to equal such standards.

Running the meeting

It is important that your meetings should always be on the same day at the same hour—if monthly, for instance, on the third Thursday at 4 pm. This allows members to reserve the time long in advance and ensures maximum attendance.

Your secretary should keep an up-to-date list of the addresses to which members of the committee wish their correspondence to be sent, and all letters and papers should invariably go by first-class post. Members should receive a letter in good time requesting submission of items for the agenda not later than three and a half weeks before the committee sits. You and your secretary must then prepare the agenda and ensure that it reaches members three weeks in advance so that its contents may be studied and any local opinions and additional information a member requires for the meeting obtained. The order of the items is important. If someone who is not a member of the committee is to attend for a particular item it should be placed first so that he or she may leave thereafter. The most important items should be taken when attendance is maximal—that is, after the late arrivals and before the early departures. Contentious issues are often best left until the end of the meeting when members will be running out of combative steam and longing for their gin and tonics.

Two or three days before the meeting you should discuss with your secretary how each item on the agenda should be handled. It is also helpful to discuss particularly difficult items informally with any member whose interests are affected or who you know holds strong views.

It is essential that you should be there to welcome members when they arrive and that you familiarise yourself with their names and background as early as possible. Tea or coffee should be provided before the meeting, which should always begin promptly at the appointed time.

No meeting should last longer than an hour and a half, preferably much less. Apart from the expenditure of time, members' concentration diminishes and they tend to drift away to other commitments. Long meetings indicate either that you are a poor chairperson or that the agenda is too long, in which case it is wise to obtain assent for an executive committee comprising yourself, the secretary and at the most two or three others to meet a few days before the main committee and deal with all the minor and uncontentious items.

At the beginning of each meeting you should welcome members, particularly newcomers, and thank them for their attendance. You should endeavour to ensure that everyone present is involved in the discussion at some time so that they may feel that they have made a contribution, and if any item has particular relevance to a member's department or special interest he or she should be invited to speak first and again before the discussion closes. At the end of the meeting you should thank members again for their attendance and provide a stirrup cup before they depart.

Follow up

The draft minutes should reach members while the proceedings are still fresh in their minds, amendments requested, and thanks for their attendance again tendered.

At the end of each year a brief letter or a Christmas card to members thanking them for their help and interest is greatly appreciated.

If everyone were invariably courteous, considerate, helpful, and unselfish, chairing a committee would be a pleasure, but they are not and after three or four meetings you will know exactly how each member will react to everything that is discussed and who dislikes whom. No one's nature or attitude will change in middle life and you can only make the best of the members you have by exercising tact, persuasion, and friendship. Your choice of a deputy chairperson is important. He or she will stand in for you if you are ill or abroad and will be one staunch ally on whom you can always rely. Some members never attend. This may be because they have another more pressing standing commitment at the same time, but it usually means that they are not interested and in such circumstances the body they represent should be informed and asked if they wish to make another nomination.

There are less rewarding activities than chairing a committee, but not many!

3 Organise a new department

S R Naik

Organising a new department is not easy. This may be because there is no formal training in the art of organising departments except in commerce and business. In this chapter I refer mainly to problems of building and organising an academic medical department. Conventionally, and sadly, the people who head departments are selected by virtue of their seniority or, sometimes, their academic background rather than their qualifications and abilities for good organisation. Senior people often crave to occupy these positions because of the attendant power but they are often not aware of the responsibilities involved. Some of them may not even realise that they are getting an opportunity to create something special.

It is true that few senior people get an opportunity to start an altogether new department. Most simply move in as departmental heads when these positions are vacated. A few of my colleagues and I got a rare opportunity of moving from our positions as heads of established departments to organise brand new departments when our new institute of selected medical specialties opened some years ago. All of us now agree that this was a challenging although difficult job. But it has allowed us to build departments that could progress fast, free of rigid systems and narrow outlooks, which often limit the potential for improving or revamping established practices.

First thoughts

If you ever decide to take up the challenge of a new department, I am sure you will subconsciously work out fresh ideas, strategies and plans. The impressions formed of the departments you have worked in or visited in the past will be recalled. You will obviously want to have a first-class department, one that will have few shortcomings and most of the merits of the other departments. Positive previous experiences will help you to entertain pleasant dreams for the future. From these images you can prepare a blueprint of your department, your own little brave new world.

Setting the goals

The first exercise you must undertake is deciding the goals of your department. There will always be some guidelines available; and yours may not be the first department of its kind. For an academic medical department you will have to consider clinical services, training, and research as the three broad goals, and you will want to set your aims high and define these goals clearly and distinctively. How do you go about this? At this stage it is worth involving selected peers and like-minded professional colleagues, some of whom you could look forward to having with you as long-term advisers and even as members of your staff. External advisers have a special importance because they can be forthright in their criticism and advice without being partisan. The key to success in the early steps in planning lies in drawing up this list of advisers who will give unflinching and genuine support to the department. It is of paramount importance to avoid choosing people whose motives are likely to clash with those of your department; it is better to have no one at all if that is the case.

As you proceed, you will, of course, acquire your own initial staff members, who should be picked because you believe them to be thoroughly dependable and capable. Once you have acquired staff and advisers to help you, you must ensure, through a process of repeated discussions and a fair exchange of views, that you all share broad aims and concepts. You will now be in a position to propose a plan for the department. A thorough planning at this stage will include outlining detailed plans of every section of the department and its functions. You will have to think in terms of reducing uncertainties to the minimum, bearing in mind that the overall plan may still need to be tailored to suit budgets imposed by the institution.

Detailed proposal

After your proposal has been submitted, it will probably be scrutinised by the relevant body. Based on its comments and questions, you may be asked for further clarifications and justifications of some of the plans. If the plans are approved with or without modifications, you may be asked to submit further detailed proposals. You may also have to give an expert opinion on issues that emerge from your special requirements. You may thus have to interact with different departments: (i) the architect for space requirement; (ii) the financial consultants for budgetary requirements; (iii) the administrators for manpower; and (iv) the stores department for technical equipment, consumables, furniture, stationery and pharmacy items, etc.

Lucky are those whose needs are mundane enough to be covered by the standard manuals provided by the state or scientific societies. If you have planned for specialised and unusual functions about which these other departments have not even the most basic understanding, you and your colleagues might have to struggle to prepare your demands in a simple step-by-step manner. You should never omit the crucial step of consulting at this stage the persons who are ultimately going to do the actual work.

After all these discussions you will be in a position to present your demands under the following headings. Your department will have certain routine and specialised *functions*; these will be performed by different people, whose numbers, qualifications, experience and other particulars you will have to project (*workforce*). These projections will enable you to indicate where these persons will physically be located (*space*) and which tools they will use (*equipment*). You will need to calculate the cost of all the above demands as the initial capital cost, add to it the running recurrent cost, and present an overall *budget proposal*.

Of the above points, functions and workforce require further discussion.

Functions

Detailing the functions of your department may be a little difficult, yet it is the most crucial and basic step, on which all other requirements depend. Two aspects merit careful consideration before you decide on this vital issue.

The first point is to decide if your department will perform specialised tasks based on certain "thrust area" programmes or whether it will be comprehensive in its functions. This may in turn depend on your area's particular needs; for example, if your centre is surrounded by several others that handle routine material, there will be little point served in your department doing the same. You should therefore carefully choose specific, well-defined areas to provide newer facilities. The selection of thrust-area programmes should be a conscious decision based on sound judgment. It is often prudent to limit and channel the development of the department and to avoid haphazard growth.

The second aspect of planning functions is that the department must be end-user stimulated. You may plan to investigate in depth patients with certain common diseases or you may want to launch selected treatment programmes. As a training organisation you need to keep in mind the requirements and aspirations of the trainee group and how your training will help them to find useful employment. As a research unit you have to plan to find answers to the questions you have decided to look at. Undoubtedly this will be a dynamic area, which will demand a flexible and adaptable approach.

Workforce planning

The department's workforce has to be planned carefully. In an academic medical department you plan for the faculty, technicians, and administrative staff. On the hospital side you will plan for nurses. There will be many other supporting staff members in other ranks that each section will need. You will have to exercise the utmost care to ensure that you have just the right number – no more and no less. Your detailed proposal for the workforce will include a full complement, but you will fill the positions in phases. This will ensure that you allocate enough time for the adaption and acclimatisation of the initial members so that a work ethic conforming to the values and aims of the department evolves smoothly.

With such scheduling you will learn more about the aptitudes, skills, strengths and weaknesses of your existing staff and determine how they fit into your thrust programmes. An appraisal of the lacunae of the department at this stage will enable you to decide on the number and the type of new members to add to the team. At this stage you will also be in a better position to specify your requirements much more precisely than ever before.

While planning for skilled workers such as technicians or specialised nurses, it is unwise to assume that they will be freely available.

It is therefore worth considering setting up your own training programmes to make up the shortfall.

Choosing the workforce

The task of finding the right kind of staff for a new department is indeed daunting, because although you will find around you many bright and talented people, some of them may have adopted negative attitudes over the years and may have lost hopes of realising their aspirations. You will therefore have to work slowly and cautiously to spot a combination of intelligence, talent, and optimism in your potential colleagues.

What is the best way to select people who are most suited to carry out particular functions? Our present system is to advertise as widely as possible throughout the general and scientific press, detailing the type of person, the desired qualifications, experience and aptitudes we are seeking, and the salaries and benefits that are offered. Details given are carefully honed to deter unnecessary applicants. Shortlisted candidates appear in front of a selection committee consisting of the head of our institution, the head of the department, and two or three of our listed advisers as experts. For key positions I strongly recommend encouraging shortlisted candidates to visit your departments before the final interview. Institutions in some countries offer positions to people on the basis of their past performance without insisting on personal interviews, but in my view this practice may not achieve the purpose of hiring the best talent. Interviews should provide the candidates and the members of the selection committee ample opportunity to talk to each other. As the head of the department you must ensure the quality of the candidates and their suitability for the particular post. The candidates must be clear about what will be expected of them. If they have to opt to limit or change their sphere of work in terms of your thrust areas, this is the time to let them know. They must also know the salary and other benefits so that successful applicants are fully satisfied at the time of entry into the department.

The image of the department

Working atmosphere

The foundation of a successful department depends a lot on a harmonious relationship and a measure of understanding among its members; these help to build an early team spirit, which can be rather difficult to inculcate later.

You might be amused to know how many trivial matters determine departmental harmony. Take the example of a new member – a staff member or trainee entering your department. He or she comes in with some apprehension, hope, or even awe. He or she naturally expects a certain type of reception, such as a warm greeting, friendly introduction to other members, familiarisation with new surroundings, and certain practical facilities, like a desk, a chair and a telephone. I know of people who have resigned soon after joining because some of these conditions had not been met. On the other hand, if you are too exuberant in your reception of a new member, older members may feel somewhat jealous. These are situations you will have to face, for which knowledge of human psychology is invaluable.

You will have to provide a sense of security and self-esteem for all your team members through education, consultation, appreciation, and other incentives. Your team members must be made to feel valuable and useful to the department to encourage a sense of belonging and pride. There will be tussles and friction among individuals and demands for more facilities, so much so that you will find it difficult to distinguish between need and greed. You will have to ensure that these problems are solved in such a way that the department emerges as a fair, just, and decent place in which to work. Opportunities for meeting informally and socially at this stage are also an important means of creating an atmosphere of cordiality, friendliness, and openness. In these ways you help to maintain and enhance the morale of your colleagues, who are the department's best ambassadors.

Public relations

Does a department need ambassadors? Whatever the debate on the issue, the answer is that you cannot function in isolation. The department shares with the institution the responsibility of service to the public and other end-users. The watchdogs of the institution's performance include the media, voluntary groups, and end-users. To an academic medical department, the end-users may be patients, students, research workers and others, who look forward to being members of your department. Points of contact with these groups and individuals must therefore be smooth and gentle. There could be many examples of these contact points – patients attending a busy outpatient clinic, students appearing at an entrance examination, or candidates facing a job interview. All these people will have variable perceptions of the likely treatment they will receive in your department. Anticipating and understanding them will enable you to provide fair and decent treatment. You must, however, ensure that these attempts at public relations are spontaneous and not contrived.

Myths and slogans

Public relations, and in equal measure, interpersonal relationships within the department, should not be based on myths and slogans about the policies of the department. Minor successes often prompt department heads to publicise vociferously their policies. Some heads project themselves as moral models for other members to emulate. Such actions are, to say the least, shortsighted and harmful to the department in the long term. They impose heavy demands on all the members to live up to the propaganda, and distract them from their real duties. It is therefore far better to keep a low profile and maintain a genuine and sincere devotion to the main activities of the department. Allow your department to be seen as human, accessible, and even vulnerable rather than mechanical, snobbish, and overefficient.

Running a new department

You will find running a new department an altogether different ball game if you have so far been looking after an established unit. Your leadership qualities will be tested as never before. You and your colleagues will be under a constant strain to continue developing the department, and you will be watched within and outside it with expectations, hope, and cynicism. The demands to perform more, quicker, and better may lead to clashes of interest and a lot of mental tension for all concerned. The key to effective running of the department in such circumstances lies in:

- the involvement and participation of all the members;
- effective decentralisation;
- development of consensus on all policy matters and difficult day-to-day problems.

It is particularly important to acknowledge the good work of your colleagues and to provide promotional avenues to people at the right moment. Stagnation of people who perform well is an early sign of malfunction of the department. If your members have to come and ask you for promotions, it could be humiliating for them and could undermine your role as leader. There may also be a difficult case of an obviously poor performer who entered the department in spite of your careful selection process. He or she will need educating, motivating, and, if these do not work, relocating and even weeding out as tactfully as possible. Harnessing and channelling the energies and talents of your gifted members and making use of others' obviously limited qualities are crucial to steering your department towards its goals.

Monitoring progress

Once you have built your department, you have to sustain its progress. You will almost certainly need to introduce at this stage some way of obtaining feedback on your performance. Your end-users—patients, trainees, volunteers for clinical research—as well as your team members, peers, and advisers have all helped you. Have all these people been asked for their views now? Are they satisfied that your department has performed well and met its goals?

The simplest way to start this type of monitoring is to keep registers for complaints, comments, and suggestions at several convenient points for your end-users and encourage them to enter their views, anonymously if they prefer. The feedback must be collated and discussed in your departmental meetings and adequate steps to redress grievances or to improve an existing service should be set in motion.

Conclusions

Organising a department is a difficult exercise, but it is a thrilling experience if you achieve your goals. Throughout this time you will, it is hoped, have learnt of your capabilities and of your weaknesses; and you will have devised your own ways of enlisting suitable help in areas where you are likely to fail. You will thus have built a human and not a mechanical organisation.

By now you will perhaps also have come to realise that there are other people, some even better than you in some respects, to whom you can hand over your proud creation when you want to retire. When you do, look back with satisfaction at what you have created, know that it is something good, but that the best is yet to come here or elsewhere.

Further reading

Bryman A. *Leadership and organization*. London: Routledge and Kegan Paul, 1986.
Brent R L. The changing role and responsibilities of chairmen in clinical academic departments, the transition from autocracy. *Pediatrics*. 1992; **90**:50–7.
Cutlip S M, Center A H. *Effective public relations*. 5th ed. New York: Prentice-Hall, 1978.
Stewart V, Stewart A. *Managing the poor performer*. London: Gower, 1988.

4 Get a patient into a mental hospital

Andrew Smith
Revised by Roderick Λ Smith and Eileen Spiller

How you get a patient into a mental hospital depends on whether or not the patient is willing to go there. If he or she is, admission is as easy as getting a physically ill patient into hospital. Telephone the hospital, describe the patient's history and symptoms to the doctor on call, and the patient will be admitted. This is informal admission and it is generally in the best interests of the patient and relatives in that it avoids the stigma of being sectioned under the Mental Health Act.

Assessment for admission under the Mental Health Act

For the patient refusing to go willingly, formal or compulsory admission has to be considered, using the Mental Health Act of 1993.[1] To invoke compulsory admission one of the following criteria has to be satisfied:

- the interests of the patient's own health, or
- the interests of the patient's own safety, or
- for the protection of other people.

Sections 2 and 3 of the Act are the ones predominantly used. Section 2 applies to a mental disorder that warrants detention in hospital for assessment (or assessment followed by medical treatment) and is for a maximum of 28 days. Pointers for using section 2 are:

- an unclear diagnosis and prognosis,

27

- a need for inpatient assessment to formulate a treatment plan,
- where a judgment is needed as to whether the patient will accept treatment voluntarily following admission,
- where a patient previously admitted under the Act is judged to have changed since the previous admission and needs further assessment,
- the patient's first admission.

Section 3 is applicable in cases of mental illness, severe mental impairment, psychopathic disorder or mental impairment of a nature or degree that makes medical treatment in hospital appropriate, and is for a maximum of six months. In the case of psychopathic disorder or mental impairment, the treatment must be likely to alleviate or prevent a deterioration of the patient's condition. Section 3 is used for an admission where the patient has been admitted in the past, is considered to need compulsory admission for the treatment of a mental disorder known to his or her clinical team, and has been assessed in the recent past by that team.

In exceptional circumstances section 4, admission for assessment in an emergency, can be used. An emergency arises where those involved cannot cope with the mental state or behaviour of the patient, and there must be evidence of the existence of a significant risk of mental or physical harm to the patient or others, the danger of serious harm to property, and/or the need for physical restraint of the patient. This requires only one doctor, usually the general practitioner, and should be used only in a genuine emergency, where an approved doctor cannot be obtained within a reasonable time.

Who is involved in a compulsory admission?

A compulsory admission involves the patient and three other people, an approved social worker and two doctors, the first approved under section 12(2) by the regional health authority, commonly a consultant psychiatrist, and the second a doctor with previous acquaintance with the patient, commonly the patient's general practitioner. Where this is not possible (for example, where the patient is not registered with a general practitioner), the second doctor should also be an approved doctor. The general practitioner is often the first person involved in a potential compulsory admission and needs to contact the approved social worker and approved doctor. Both should be available on 24-hour rotas.

Formal application for admission has to be made by either an approved social worker or the nearest relative, preferably the former, who, once contacted, is responsible for overall coordination of the assessment and admission process. Normally, the social worker will see the patient alone, but may insist on the presence of another professional where he or she fears physical harm. Where direct access to the patient is not immediately possible, there are powers in the Act to secure access (section 135), and the police can be asked to see if they would exercise lawful power of entry. The patient may request a friend's presence at the interview. The social worker should attempt to identify the nearest relative and is statutorily required to inform him or her of an application under section 2 or 3.

The doctors need to examine the patient together where practical, but if they do this separately, they should always discuss the patient with each other. At least one doctor, but preferably both need to discuss the patient with the applicant. Where the two doctors have jointly examined the patient, forms 3 and 10 can be used, and should be completed and signed by both doctors at the same time; in all other circumstances separate recommendation forms (forms 4 and 11) should be used. The approved doctor needs to ensure that a hospital bed is available.

The approved social worker is responsible for arranging transfer to hospital and ensuring that the correctly completed admission documents arrive at hospital at the same time as the patient. The patient will usually be sent by ambulance, but may be sent by private car if the social worker is satisfied that the patient will not be a danger to himself/herself or others. If the patient is likely to be violent or dangerous, the police should be asked to help. The patient should never be sent in a private car without an escort in addition to the driver.

1 *Code of practice Mental Health Act 1983*. London: Department of Health and Welsh Office, 1993.

5 Be a dictator

Heather Windle

Despite the proliferation of word processors and computers capable of handling routine letters, doctors still find it necessary to dictate one-off letters, papers, reports, and so on. Word processors, incidentally, have dangers: a sentence may carelessly be changed without the rest of the text being checked for inconsistencies, and mistakes are often repeated ad infinitum. It is as well to remember that a computer lacks imagination and its brain is limited by the quality of the data fed in by the operator. Even so, they are addictive and many a doctor has become hooked on a computer.

However, this does not mean that doctors will type their own letters; they will undoubtedly need someone else to cope with correspondence and papers, but I hope they will use their computers for referral and recall letters, letters to insurance companies and employers so that they can make the best use of their secretaries or shorthand or audio typists.

A few doctors have mentioned to me how inadequate they feel when confronted by an efficient-looking woman or, less usually, man with a notebook and a pencil poised, expectantly waiting for them to begin speaking. What can they do to overcome their nervousness, they ask. No doubt the answer is to have confidence in their knowledge about the matter to be dictated, but they seem to be more concerned about technique. I may be able to help because during a particularly horrendous period in my life when my children were at school I worked as a temporary secretary for some 200-300 different men (99% *were* men, but with equal opportunities for all no doubt the percentage has gone down, particularly in the medical world).

During that time I encountered practically every good and bad type of personality imaginable, and every possible vagary in typewriter, tape-recorder, and other machines, for which I had little natural aptitude. My sympathies, therefore, are primarily with the person on the receiving end of dictation, but I admit to a little experience on the other side of the fence, which was almost as difficult because I was young at the time and my secretary was old.

You may dictate direct or into a dictating machine or tape-recorder, and both have advantages and disadvantages. If you are doing it by remote control—for example, a consultant who goes to a hospital once a week, dictates into a machine, and signs the finished letters a week later—then presumably you will continue on this antisocial course. If you dictate direct or have any other communication with the secretary or shorthand or audio typist, however, please call her (even nowadays it is usually a woman) by her name—let's say it is Jane—and treat her as if she is as clever, or almost as clever, as you. She won't be a doctor but, unknown to you, may have a first in English or an IQ of 140; she will be more willing to stop you making mistakes if you take advantage of at least some of her talents. You may both find a mixture of shorthand and dictating machine the best way to manage work that may be dictated during office hours or outside them.

Jane should be able to write some letters herself if you give her a rough outline of what you want to say. Let her do as much as she is capable of, because that will retain her interest better than routine dictation. If you treat her well she will do much for you—as well as correcting your grammar, she may remind you about unanswered or forgotten letters, or point out mistakes you are making in other ways. A great deal, however, will have to be done by dictation.

Shorthand

Shorthand has great advantages. You or Jane can correct letters easily as you go along or afterwards if they are longwinded or rubbish, and Jane can tell you when you've repeated yourself. Make sure she has a suitable chair and a word processor that works properly. She may be nervous, so collect your thoughts and the day's work together (if possible, dictate in one or two batches, but not for too long at a stretch, and then leave her in peace), and, if you are a muddler, make a few notes to guide you, and give the notes to Jane when you've finished. You should be able to judge the best speed to dictate by whether Jane looks frantic or bored—in time, her speed will increase to match yours, but take it easy to start with. If you can restrain yourself, punctuate only when essential, because punctuation distracts, and you shouldn't have to make her read the whole thing back.

When answering letters give Jane the originals and do not dictate the address. Spell out difficult words—drugs and diseases, for example—and don't say "Dear Jumbo" without indicating who he is. Correcting typed letters in ink was maddening in the days of typewriters, but not a problem with the ubiquitous word processor as long as your handwriting is legible—not a virtue all doctors can claim! You should take advantage of your contact with her. If you want her to stay on, ask her sometimes for her opinion. She will be flattered and you may be surprised to find that she has useful ideas about speeches and articles.

Recording problems

One snag about recording is that people tend to like the sound of their own voices, letters become prolix, and addressees merely scan them and perhaps miss the point. So keep the letters short, and do give Jane an idea of the length. Another snag is second thoughts; nothing is more irritating than to hear half way through: "Sorry, scrub the first paragraph". No one wants to waste time and energy doing useless work. You can easily erase the tape and start again. Remember, too, that Jane will first have to type the letters exactly as she hears them, if she is a typist only, so don't be surprised if they are returned to you looking like the writings of an illiterate schoolboy; and if she is a secretary or personal assistant, she will need to take additional time putting them into reasonable shape —she has little chance of correcting them as she plays the tape. Another, and more serious, snag is the time it takes for an overworked audiotypist to tackle a tape. Once you have dictated something it's easy to forget that it hasn't come back for signature. This hardly ever happens with shorthand.

Many secretaries prefer to be separated from their bosses by machines, but there is still room for the personal touch. If you mention Jane's name on the tape sometimes, if only to say "Good morning, Jane", or "Jane, please remind me about that", it makes all the difference to a good working partnership, but fatuous remarks about the test match or the weather go down less well.

Points to remember

Dictating in the street, car, nursery, plane, or train makes transcribing difficult for Jane when she has to sort out your words from children's cries, traffic sounds, or Bach.

If you and Jane have different mother tongues or idioms (Americans can be as difficult as Greeks or Romans), dictate slowly and, if necessary, repeat words with a different emphasis—otherwise the words will still be double Dutch to her. If you can't spell, employ someone who can (have a list of words to try out on her), or you may become the object of ridicule—my daughter and a publisher boss of hers sent out hundreds of letters about "soul distribution rights" before they were spotted. And don't wander away from the microphone or hold it at greatly varying distances from your mouth while you are dictating: either chunks will be missing from your letters, or Jane will go mad trying to adjust the volume before being deafened.

One word about speeches: write down an outline before dictating, because you may lose the thread, and give the notes to Jane. Normally, you should be willing to answer her questions (better for her to ask than get it wrong), but with a speech she may be reluctant to interrupt you.

There are other ways of dictating, most of them torture. You may dictate to Jane over the telephone and not visualise her desk covered in papers, another telephone ringing, people interrupting her, and her neck getting a cramp as she tries to balance the receiver on her shoulder so that her hands are free to take down your vital words. If you must do that, make sure Jane's telephone has a speaker monitor that allows her to hear calls without lifting the receiver.

I have concentrated on how to be a dictator and omitted the more subtle secretarial side of Jane's job, but, whether she is a secretary or a typist, you should treat her with patience and consideration, talk *with* her sometimes rather than at her, and don't treat her as if she is half witted. If you're nice to her, she'll put up with you when you are occasionally irritable, forgetful, unreasonable, or overbearing. Remember, it's not *fun* taking down your dictation, it's a job, so try to make the job as interesting for her as you can. If you trust her—and you should not employ her if you don't—you may even be able to grant her access to your computer files with a codeword of her own: then she will be able to handle some of the data more accurately than you do and also be spared some of the drudgery of her own work.

6 Dictate a discharge summary

T M Penney

The main communication that a general practitioner receives about his or her patient's admission to hospital is the formal typed hospital discharge summary. This forms the core of available information and as such is of vital importance. Unfortunately, the task of dictating this summary is often regarded as a chore by the hospital doctor, which need not be the case if the job is tackled in a logical, systematic way.

At present there is a delay of about three weeks before the general practitioner receives the discharge summary.[1-3] The reasons for the delay are various but probably include delays in dictation and typing and postal delays.[1] If the summary can be dictated sooner, and in a way that requires the minimum of secretarial time, benefits will be reaped in several ways: the hospital doctor will enjoy up-to-date notes, the general practitioner will be aware of his or her patient's condition sooner, and the patients will be able to discuss their hospital stay and all its implications with their family doctor. Currently the system fails us.

I describe here how to dictate a discharge summary based on my own experiences and observations. I see no reason why most discharge summaries should not be received by the general practitioner within seven days of the patient's discharge if my guidelines are followed. With a standard format and better organisation the service can be vastly improved. It really is very easy to produce documents containing concise, relevant information if the right attitude to the task is adopted.

The advent of the purchaser/provider split, and of general

```
Dr Smith                                                          Date
The Surgery
Anytown

Dear Dr Smith,
                    Re: Arthur BEST, 123 Anyroad, Anytown
                         Date of birth 1 2 34
                         Hospital No 567890

Admitted

Discharged

Diagnosis

History

Past medical history

Medication on admission

Examination

Investigations

Treatment and progress

Medication on discharge

Follow up

Yours sincerely

Dr Jones

Senior house officer to Dr Brown, consultant
```

Fig 1 Standard discharge summary

practitioner fundholding, has given further emphasis to the provision of accurate data from hospitals. Funds are paid to providers based upon what happened to the patient while in hospital, with the clinical discharge letter holding the basic information for each admission. Inaccurate or missing clinical information may confound monetary disputes.

Design

I propose that all discharge summaries should be typed in one of two basic formats (figs 1 and 2). This would simplify the secretary's task and doctors would soon become accustomed to the design, so minimising the chance of any important details being omitted. Standard formats have been used successfully before.[4]

35

Dr Smith   Date
The Surgery
Anytown

Dear Dr Smith

Re: Arthur BEST, 123 Anyroad, Anytwown
Date of birth 1 2 34
Hospital No 567890

Your patient underwent a routine   operation on
. There were no complications and he was discharged on
, with the following medication: . Please arrange for
removal of stitches in   days. Follow up will not/will be arranged for
weeks.

Yours sincerely

Dr Jones

Senior house officer to Dr Brown, consultant

Fig 2 Short discharge letter

The short discharge letter may be used for any routine admission that is not complicated, when the general practitioner does not need detailed information. It lends itself especially to patients who have had operations and it can be adapted to suit each particular admission. To stick rigidly to a detailed format for a routine appendicectomy, for example, wastes time and effort.

For most admissions the standard discharge summary can be used. Some of the sections, however, could be omitted in certain cases—for instance, "Past medical history", "Medication on admission", and perhaps even "Examination" and "Investigations". The general practitioner does not really need to know that "there were signs of consolidation at the right base posteriorly and a consolidated area in the chest radiograph" if the diagnosis of pneumonia of the right lower lobe is written at the top of the page.

Details

The details written under each heading in the discharge summary should be concise and relevant. Strictly speaking, only details relevant to the general practitioner to whom the letter is addressed should be included. The copy of the summary left in the hospital notes, however, can be extremely useful to a subsequent admitting

36

doctor because it acts as a précis of past events. For this reason some hospital practitioners will prefer, for instance, to give negative results of investigations as well as positive ones in the summary. I contend that to keep summaries as short as possible, and therefore save as much time as possible, such details should be omitted. It takes only a few seconds to turn to the investigation sheets in the hospital notes. A short, relevant, and concise summary is much more likely to be read through by a busy general practitioner than a long letter full of irrelevant material.

The most important headings for the general practitioner are "Diagnosis", "Medication on discharge", and "Follow-up". In cases in which a new diagnosis has been made a few details under an additional heading of "Information given to the patient" would be invaluable. Awkward situations have arisen when patients have not been given vital pieces of information that the general practitioner has taken for granted and misunderstandings have subsequently occurred.

When each senior house officer takes up a new post the consultant should go over the system of discharge summaries used in the department and give initial guidance on the standards expected.

Dictation

Now that a standard format has been designed and the information condensed, time must be found to dictate the summary. In my experience no specific time is set aside for a senior house officer to dictate summaries. The time must be found during the course of an already busy day, and this is often after everyone else has gone home. I well remember spending hours sitting alone in a darkened office, occasionally interrupted by the cleaner. Many senior house officers take their work home with them, although this is not wise because of the problems that arise concerning the security and confidentiality of patients' notes when they are taken outside the hospital.

Time should be made available every week—30 minutes should be sufficient—to dictate summaries. Perhaps the best time would be after the main ward round of the week, when decisions about discharging patients tend to be taken. Summaries could be dictated when the patients are sent home; the document will reach the general practitioner sooner, and the patients' individual details will be fresh in the mind of the senior house officer. Thus important

37

details are less likely to be omitted and a better summary will be produced. If summaries are not dictated for several weeks it becomes more difficult to put a face to the patient's name. One has to thumb through notes to find the relevant information rather than being able to dictate most of the summary direct from memory.

I have experienced several disincentives to dictate summaries, the main one being a huge pile of notes overflowing from my pigeon hole in the consultant's office. A backlog develops surprisingly quickly, particularly at the start of a new hospital job. Often the senior house officer changes every six months, and the outgoing doctor may leave a residue of undictated notes behind. This is a dirty trick and quite unforgivable. The temptation would not be so great if dictation were performed promptly throughout the period of the job. Locums who do not dictate summaries on patients they look after present another problem; perhaps allocating the next senior member of the team to do the summaries while the senior house officer is away would help matters. A similar system could be adopted to cover holidays.

Equipment can also be a problem. Doctors should check that their dictaphones are recording properly and that their tapes are not damaged. I once came to the end of a long dictating session and checked the tape, only to find that the whole recording had been reduced to a series of unintelligible whirring and grinding noises.

Dispatch

After the summary has been dictated, the tape should be labelled, attached to the notes, and left in a prearranged place for the secretary. Unfortunately, there is a general shortage of medical secretaries at present,[5] and typing may take several days or weeks. The senior house officer should make a habit of visiting the secretary's office regularly to sign the documents when they have been typed so that they may be posted without delay. Many hospitals use second-class post.

1 Penney T M. Delayed communications between hospitals and general practitioners: where does the problem lie? *BMJ* 1988; **297**: 28–9.
2 Mageean R J. Study of "discharge communications" from hospital. *BMJ* 1986; **293**: 1283–4.
3 Tulloch A J, Fowler G H, McMillan J J, Spence J M. Hospital discharge reports: content and design. *BMJ* 1975; iv: 443–6.
4 Stevenson J G, Murray Boyle C, Alexander W D. A new hospital discharge letter. *Lancet* 1973; i: 928–31.
5 Miller H C. Delayed communication between hospitals and general practitioners. *BMJ* 1988; **297**: 292.

7 Design a clinical information system

A P Smith

When in 1989 my department decided to get a clinical information system we quickly realised that we would have to do it ourselves. Everything we looked at was much too expensive and very complicated. Three years and many workhours later our clinical information system, Dossier, was up and running. The system won the personal computer rewards competition sponsored by the Peat Marwick group and the *Guardian* in November 1991. This paper describes the key points we learnt, which should be taken into account when planning a clinical information system.

Dossier is a real time, episode based, clinical information system designed around the daily work of the medical secretary. Clinical data are collected as discharge summaries and outpatient letters are typed, although on a networked system remote workstations could be used to record the presence of a patient, the secretary doing the rest while typing the discharge summary. Because our system is real time, information is immediately available to other users as it is entered, and as it is episode based and records activity as it happens, it gives an accurate picture of workload.

Who will enter data?

Before starting this project our knowledge of computers was limited to the usual experience of anyone doing clinical research— word processing, simple databases, medical statistics, and so on. But designing and writing this type of computer programme is as much about attitudes and philosophy as technique, and the ground rules are simple.

The fewer the people who enter information and the smaller the dataset, the more likely you are to get a full and accurate record on every case. Our dataset (see table) is clinically determined and omits items such as provider and purchaser codes, overseas visitor status, NHS number, place of birth, occupation of spouse and parent, discharge method, and destination. The choice was determined entirely by availability (who knows their NHS number?) and potential usefulness to clinicians, although we are going to have to include some of the items we originally left out because managers will need them.

When deciding on a dataset, you will have to compromise between ease of data entry and demands for all sorts of information, but it is best to exclude information that is difficult to collect. Unfortunately, many recommended datasets are so inflated that no clinical department will ever be able to collect them. It should take no longer to enter a new patient and code into the computer than it takes a secretary to write the letters now, so resist unreasonable pressure to include unnecessary or awkward data items—they simply do not get filled in, or, if compulsory, slow the process of data entry to the point that it becomes irksome.

How will data be validated?

Consider how you will validate the contents of your database. Dossier saves the name of the person who last used a record so we know who is responsible for its accuracy. Because key items of information in the database appear in letters and summaries, validation takes place when these are signed, and the signatory is responsible for that patient's record. The programme also checks for obvious errors, such as patients getting discharged before they are admitted, and will not permit the user to exit a screen until all essential items are entered correctly. Dossier comes with an archive utility to store defunct records on a floppy disk and a range of other utilities, including hard-disk back-up and restore. Most users would probably prefer to use a tape streamer for back-ups, especially as the size of the database increases, and this would be essential on a networked system.

Data held on Dossier clinical information system

Field	How information is stored (No. of characters)	Validation
Data held on every patient:		
Name	Character (30)	Valid if not empty
Hospital number	Alphanumeric (8)	By user. Non obligatory
Address	Character (60)	Valid if not empty
Postcode	Character (8)	Valid if not empty
Telephone number	Character (12)	By user. Non obligatory
Sex	Logical (1)	Valid M/F
Referral type	Character (2)	Valid if not empty. User defined, entry from pop up table of 6 choices
Alive or dead	Logical (1)	Valid if not empty
In or out status	Logical (1)	Valid if not empty
Date of birth	Date (8)	Date validation
Date first seen	Date (8)	Date validation
Date admitted or attended clinic	Date (8)	Date validation
Date discharged or died	Date (8)	Date validation
General practitioner number	Numeric (5)	Created by system
Unique patient identification	Numeric (5)	Created by system. Relational key
Archived flag	Logical (1)	Created by system
Data held when available:		
Diagnosis	Character (76)	Text entered by medical secretary from dictation
Treatment	Character (152)	Text entered from dictation
Action	Character (20)	Follow up, waiting list, etc
Last seen by	Character (20)	Name of doctor seeing patient
Codes	Character (76)	List of codes generated by coding utility
Text field	Character (64 000)	Full word processor. Contains text for letter
Last altered by	Character (20)	Automatically entered with user's passname if record altered
Length of stay	Numeric (3)	Days calculated and entered automatically
Cumulative outpatient count	Numeric (3)	Counts number of outpatient episodes
Cumulative inpatient count	Numeric (3)	Counts number of inpatient episodes

Note: Users can design and subsequently select and enter a full screen of data, which can be disease, specialty or audit dependent, at each clinical transaction. Serial numerical items from these records may be displayed in tables or graphs against time.

Will the system overburden staff?

Think of your secretary. You will get no extra staff to run your computer. No system should increase secretaries' workloads; instead it should make them more efficient and happy. The most important person is the one who puts the data in, and, like it or not, that will be somebody in your office, maybe even you. Collecting information is boring and disruptive, so you need to make it agreeable, and there must be an immediate and perceptible benefit. Medical secretaries are the primary beneficiaries of our system, the audit and managerial data are its byproducts. The system's useful features include automatically remembering and typing general practitioners' names and addresses, a word processor, interactive diagnostic and procedure coding, a "quick patient look up" facility, and a cache of every letter ever written on any patient, which is useful if the notes go missing; the system simultaneously stores the information clinicians and managers need. While these features help the secretaries in their work, they ensure accuracy too.

Use local skills

Maximise on the local clinical experience. Members of information technology committees should ferret out clinicians in their district who have already set up their own systems, and there are a lot of them about. It is important that their experience and enthusiasm be harnessed and spread to their colleagues because the idea that data collection and validation are as much part of clinical work as outpatient clinics or theatre has not generally caught on. Most doctors think it will all be done by someone else, but most of the work will be in doctors' offices, so be sure that a proposed system has been well and truly tested by real doctors and that it is acceptable in the clinical setting. Designing your own system ensures complete acceptability, of course, but not everyone will want to repeat our experience.

Big computers are to be avoided. Mainframe or mini-based applications are expensive and specialists are needed to keep them going. Installing personal computers is the cheapest way. At only a few hundred pounds they are cheap enough to throw away if they stop working, and their programming tools are inexpensive and can be used by ordinary people. We chose dBASE, got the ideas working, then switched to Clipper 5, which is less friendly but more powerful. Doctors and secretaries were involved early on and a working program containing all the essential features was put into daily use. Later, we employed a computing student from the University of Sussex during his vacations to provide the special expertise. Your solutions should avoid the need for expensive hardware and software engineers. You will always want to add new features or modifications, as it is impossible to plan a computer system in detail from scratch, and it should be possible to add these locally without great expense. The idea that you can have a cheap clinical information system running on personal computers is perfectly tenable provided that you keep it simple and decide what you really want.

Don't be overambitious

Keep to essentials and do not try to do things that can be done better or more cheaply another way. A clinical information system collects clinical data, gives you reports, and recalls patients for audit. Ours also stores all the old letters and case summaries and does the coding. Don't ask it to do anything else. The number of data items required for these purposes is quite small and so this is ideal for personal computers. One reason that existing commercial systems are so expensive is that they are too big and do too much.

Consider installing single-user systems. Although low tech, this solution encourages people in the habit of data collection and very quickly puts the means to do so on their desks. There can be few circumstances when a clinician would want to have direct access to a colleague's clinical database, and there is no reason for managers to have that privilege either; if the database is located in the consultant's office, ownership and data security are assured. As long as the information is being collected, it doesn't really matter where it is kept. Single-user systems could be on every consultant's desk for less than £3000 each, including hardware; the most expensive single item would be a good printer. In these terms it is incredible that all hospital doctors do not have this facility now; the reason they do not is that single-user systems are not interesting to managers. Once we had started using Dossier we also soon wanted to share data on a departmental basis. We compromised on our reluctance to let the data leave the consultant's office and wrote a networked departmental version, but this is as big as it should get—any bigger and costs rise, with diminishing returns.

Of course, some managers and most information technology advisors would prefer a single hospital clinical database, but their perceptions of the advantages, and the resulting costs, have slowed the introduction of systems for everyday clinical use, and it places too much power in the information technology manager's hands. Naturally, managers must have the information, but they do not need direct access to a clinical database to collect it. At the simplest level a floppy disk sent in the internal mail to put on the administration's computer each week would achieve the same object; a networked poll of departmental databases is better but is considerably more expensive. In our hospital, management has been supportive in installing clinical systems but so far has shown little interest in developing them on a hospital-wide basis. This will come, however, and future projects for Dossier include a suite of management functions that will be able to collect information from departmental databases across a hospital network.

Single-user or departmental solutions have many advantages. Everything stops when a hospital or district computer breaks down, so it needs elaborate back-up and maintenance arrangements; it is inconvenient if a smaller system fails, but life goes on. Personal computer databases can be read, copied, analysed, and manipulated by all sorts of tools, so you are not locked into any particular application and can change if anything better comes along. The simpler they are though, the greater the risk of unauthorised access, which of course is another argument for keeping it on the consultant's desk.

Build in flexibility

By now our intentions will be obvious: to free clinical users from the constraints of cost, computer experts, managers, and those who think they know best. Such freedom is essential to independent people whose data requirements vary widely. A system that imposes on or interferes with daily life will not be tolerated for long, and if the system is only tolerated, it cannot be relied on. We believe that clinicians, whose data requirements inevitably differ, must be able to decide what they want to collect within the limits of a common dataset. Our system contains screens whose functions are defined by the user on setting up for the first time, and experience has shown that we could possibly do with more.

Reporting also needs to be flexible because most people don't know the questions they will want to ask. We designed a flexible report builder that is simple enough for doctors and their secretaries to use. It allows you just to browse, which helps to formulate ideas about disease patterns—for example, the incidence of asthma referrals from a particular postal district. Alternatively, it can report in lists, synopses (statistical reviews showing subsidiary diagnoses, age and sex breakdown, referral types, and source), episode audits (statistics of inpatient and outpatient episodes with length of stay), and counts according to any item, or combination of items, in the database subject to logical analysis. To be really useful a system must permit clinicians to get at their own information whenever they like and play with it.

Benefits of the system

So we can now audit our work, wards, and clinic, and the work of juniors. We have reduced the numbers of ineffective follow-up appointments and we discharge patients earlier. For the first time, because of smaller clinics, we can run a proper appointments system; this was an unexpected bonus and the first benefit we noticed. We can investigate the causes of repeat follow-up visits and of readmissions, and by relating procedures to diagnosis and length of admission we can assess the use of resources per case.

Computers are great at assessing the use of resources, comparing workloads, treatments, and patterns of work, but is this really clinical audit? To clinicians, audit means the examination of practices, modifying them, and reviewing them later to ensure that modifications have been followed and are effective. If you cannot recall information about your patients, you cannot audit them, and in this sense computers are useful in clinical audit. But otherwise they are not required. Doctors must be clear about this. Clinical information systems contain a relatively small dataset on a large number of patients. By contrast audit needs a lot of information, which varies from audit to audit, on a subset of patients; until the audit is planned, the data to be collected are not known. So do not harbour unreasonable expectations about the role of computers in audit. A surgeon might collect data about wound infection rates, and his system could list the patients concerned, but why they got infected and what action should be taken is something he must decide for himself. All the computer can do is identify the patients for study.

45

Limit the computers' functions

One reason that computers are not generally available to hospital doctors is the impression that they must do everything—audit, office automation, management functions, case mix, keep the waiting lists, and so on. Do not fall into this trap; if you do, you will never get your system. Keep it simple, adopt an evolutionary stance, and make sure that clinical and secretarial needs are met first. Remember, too, that a clinical database requires a cultural shift which is greater than most doctors understand. It means pride in owning the data, confidence in its validity, freedom to explore and understand it, and an absence of computer bureaucracy. Of course not all doctors are interested in information technology, and you may be content with whatever comes along. But never underestimate the disruptive potential of a computer.

By doing it ourselves we learnt a lot about audit, coding, and data collection. It took three years, about the same commitment as a major clinical research project, and cost about £6000. There is not an existing system at the price. Unless a lot of new money is made available most hospital doctors will not get computers for clinical use within the reasonable future. But why wait for your information technology advisory committee to buy you a white elephant? Cheap, practical systems are available now: get started, get the experience, feel the enthusiasm grow, and you will then be able to talk to the specialists on equal terms. Who knows, you may be able to inject some clinical commonsense into the tangled world of hospital information technology.

8 Produce a service specification

Diana Webster

Since 1 April 1991 contracts have formed the basis of all NHS provisions.[1] These contracts must identify the quality, quantity, and cost of services to be provided. Before a contract can be developed, a service specification is needed.[2] Many district health authorities invited would-be providers to submit service specifications for the services they wished the health authority to purchase. In this context a service specification is an offer to provide a service.

That experience with contracts showed that provider units found it difficult to describe the services they wanted to offer in a way that was meaningful and useful to a district health authority purchaser. Clinicians are expected to participate in developing service specifications.[3] To help doctors to draw up service specifications I have identified the information a prospective purchaser needs to get maximum value from a specification.

What is a service specification?

A service specification is an offer to provide a service. It is made by a provider to a prospective purchaser. A service specification is therefore not the same as a specialty plan.

While examining a service specification the purchaser considers two fundamental questions: Do I wish to buy this service and do I wish to buy it from this particular provider? It is therefore in the interests of both parties that every specification attempts to give sufficient information to assist prospective purchasers in their deliberations.

The specification should provide sufficient information to allow the purchaser to answer five important questions: What is the service, how is it to be provided, how much service is being offered, what is the quality of the service, and can the provider deliver the quality of service promised? I will address each of these questions separately. The list of information to be included is not intended to be exhaustive and should be extended when this seems appropriate to the particular service.

What is the service being offered?

The specification should include, firstly, the overall aim of the service. For example, the overall aim of a general surgical service might be to provide comprehensive general surgical care to all patients aged 16 years and above referred in need of general surgical treatment.

Secondly, the specific objectives of the service should be stated. In a general surgical service these might include prompt assessment of acutely ill patients by a doctor with appropriate experience and training, provision of timely and appropriate operative care by adequately skilled and supervised medical staff, provision of care by doctors who are personally participating in comprehensive medical audit of the care they provide, and effective communication between medical and nursing staff and patients (and their general practitioner).

Thirdly, a description of the service is needed. This should include the range of clinical activities encompassed by the service, the specialist interests and expertise; the modes of treatment (inpatient, outpatient, day care, etc), the input from other medical and paramedical specialties (pathology, anaesthesia, physiotherapy, social work, etc), the relation and communication with services provided by other provider units (such as community child health services, community nursing, social services), the access to the service (consultant, general practitioner, non-medical health professional, self-referral, restrictions or prerequisites for treatment), and the provider's involvement in teaching, training, and research.

How is the service provided, and by whom?

Purchasers need to know the type and location of facilities. What are they? Are they good, and if so, why? What, if any, are the facilities for parents or relatives to stay overnight? What are the facilities for visitors?

The philosophy underpinning the staffing of the service should also be described. Is it a consultant-based service? If so, what is the provider's interpretation of consultant-based and how is 24-hour consultant cover maintained (especially when consultants have commitments on more than one site)? Are staff with particular expertise and qualifications employed (for example, with specialist training in intensive or paediatric care)? What are the policies for continuing within service education and updating of staff in all disciplines?

Relevant policies or codes of practice, or both, concerning the way care is provided are also important, and include, for example, policies concerning the supervision of junior staff; communication with patients, relatives, other medical or paramedical staff, etc; and individual nursing care programmes for patients. Any clinical protocols or policies should also be included (for postoperative pain relief; rehabilitation of patients with fractured neck of femur; prescribing and management of myocardial infarction, head injuries, stroke, and deliberate self harm), as should use of day surgery, five-day wards, and a planned investigation facility.

What quantity of service does the provider expect the purchaser's residents to require?

Activity data relating to residents of the purchasing district health authority are required. For example, data on episodes of inpatient care and length of stay (elective and acute); outpatient, day, and domiciliary care, and readmission rates; relevant activity data for procedures (number of hip replacements, child development assessments, etc). The specification should also include an analysis of trends and an analysis of waiting list and waiting times, and of performance over the preceding 12 months—for example, mean and range of waiting times for admission for elective surgery during the past 12 months.

What is the quality of the service being offered?

The purchaser needs objective information to explain why providers believe their service is of good quality. Information should be provided on the effectiveness, efficiency, equity, acceptability, accessibility, and appropriateness of the service being offered.

Purchasers also look for specific standards set and response to quality issues the authority has identified as priorities for the contract period.

Will the provider deliver the stated quality of service?

To assess this, purchasers look at proposals for monitoring the quality of service, in particular whether both process and outcome of care are monitored. Information on how the provider intends to implement and monitor quality standards the provider has set is also considered.

When medical audit is being practised, purchasers consider whether the provider has identified any recent changes that have been prompted by the findings of medical audit and look for details of the medical audit programme to be implemented during the next 12 months. Specifically, are the topics for audit identified and are the standards being used within the audit identified?

Finally, the purchaser considers whether the provider has confirmed that it intends to comply with the district health authority's targets and quality standards and if so how it intends to achieve compliance and monitor its performance.

The format of a service specification is a matter for discussion with individual purchasing district health authorities. Nevertheless, if providers covered the above topics this would help to reduce purchasers' concerns about the content of these specifications.

1 NHS Management Executive. *Contracts for health services: operating contracts*. London: HMSO, 1990.
2 NHS Management Executive. *Starting specifications: a DHA project paper*. London: NHS Management Executive, 1990. (EL.90:161.)
3 NHS Management Executive. *Involving professional staff in drawing up NHS contracts*. London: NHS Management Executive, 1990. (EI.90:221.)

9 Apply for charitable status

Maurice Slevin, Patsy Ryan

Creating a unique nationwide information service for patients with cancer wasn't Dr Vicky Clement-Jones's only unusual achievement when she founded the British Association of Cancer United Patients (BACUP) in 1984; she also gave a new twist to the old adage "charity begins at home", as most of the groundwork was done from her home in London while she was convalescing after treatment for advanced ovarian cancer. As her plans gathered momentum she and willing colleagues were caught up in the frantic merry-go-round of raising funds, forging contacts, and generally securing a place in the hearts (and pockets) of philanthropic money makers.

Vicky seized all opportunities with characteritic spirit and vigour, and her inspiring enthusiasm (coupled with a sense of true urgency, as her prognosis was uncertain) led to the association being registered as a charity in just three days. The year 1984 certainly had its fair share of unique achievements.

Do you register?

If your organisation is to be regarded as a charity and comes within the jurisdiction of the British High Court (which it does if it has property in England or Wales, or most of the people legally responsible for it usually live in England or Wales), it must be registered with the Charity Commissioners for England and Wales. In fact, the organisation's trustees have a legal duty to apply to the Commissioners for registration. There are some exceptions to this law; the Commissioners will be able to advise you.

51

The major advantage of registration is financial. The great British public is reassured by the respectability of a registered charity number when being persuaded to part with hard-earned cash. Even if you don't envisage rattling collecting tins at Saturday afternoon shoppers, when you are appealing to benevolent business and charitable foundations the magic number proves an effective "open sesame" to their coffers. More pragmatically, registered charities are automatically entitled to tax and ratings relief, and opportunities for donations free of tax gild the carrot to tempt valuable regular donors.

The commonest drawbacks to attaining charitable status are the strict legal limitations imposed on political and campaigning activities. This is sensitive territory, and if planning to venture into it you would be well advised to have the guiding hand of a good lawyer at your elbow. Your best guide is generally a solicitor experienced in all aspects of forming charities. The increasingly complex charity laws are a specialist subject, and experts tend to be thin on the ground. The National Council for Voluntary Organisations[1] is willing to advise on specific aspects of forming a charity.

Paths paved with charitable intentions

British law recognises four distinct categories of charitable purposes. So, unfortunately, however worthy the intentions of your future organisation, the law (and therefore charitable status) will remain impervious unless you can slot your aims neatly into one of these categories:

- relief of poverty,
- advancement of eduction,
- advancement of religion,
- specific other purposes beneficial to the community.

It is important to emphasise that any purpose cannot be charitable in law unless it is for the public benefit. That means it is of actual benefit, and benefits the public as a whole, or a significant section of the public.

Hand in hand with advice from your legal mentor on how to satisfy the legal criteria of these categories should go the principle of saving time and resources: "Never reinvent the wheel." When BACUP had little more substance than a pipe dream Vicky embarked on a fact-finding mission to the United States National

Cancer Institute. She returned with two suitcases crammed full of invaluable anecdotal advice and experience.

Building the empire

The written governing document of a charity should define the purposes and powers of the organisation and agree the means of achieving them to avoid disputes at a later date. As this worthy document is also one of the chief components of the application for registration as a charity it is worth investing time and effort to make it absolutely accurate.

Fortunately, plagiarism of a model document is acceptable— even advisable—if the chosen model fits your aims like a glove. Model governing documents for three basic types of charity are available from the Charity Commissioners for England and Wales. Otherwise, try asking a similar organisation if you can see their document.

You will need a lawyer or legal advice to guide you towards the best structure for your fledgling charity. The three main types of charity are trusts, unincorporated associations, and companies. Briefly, a trust is governed by a trust deed or will and the trustees alone are responsible for managing the organisation. An unincorporated association is probably the best structure for a group of like-minded people who want to cooperate to achieve a specified objective. The association is then governed by a written constitution or rules. Charities can also be incorporated under the Companies Act 1985 as companies limited by guarantee without a share capital. In this case the governing document is the Memorandum and Articles of Association. Companies have the main advantage of being considered as legal persons in their own right, which reduces the sometimes risky personal liabilities of trustees. BACUP began as a trust and became a company limited by guarantee when it had become firmly established.

The grand launch

The blessing of new organisations with charitable status has been firmly in the hands of the Charity Commissioners for England and Wales since 1960. The registration procedure is fairly straightforward, but usually takes some time to complete. All applicants must fill out a questionnaire from the Commissioners and send them their proposed governing document. The Commissioners consider all the information and may contact the Inland Revenue to allow it to register any objections. Once the Commissioners are satisfied that the organisation and its activities are charitable, they will invite the applicants to complete their governing document and formally apply for registration.

The Commissioners have various powers over registered charities, which include seeing regular accounts statements and being informed of changes to the governing document or registered details. All charities with an annual income of more than £5000 must state that the organisation is a registered charity on all paperwork appealing for funds and various other financial documents.

The Commissioners produce a helpful leaflet on registering charities called *Starting a Charity* (HMSO CC21).

Founding a charity is the perfect chance of a lifetime to etch your own lasting design on history's slate. Perhaps Vicky's example of starting BACUP with just one person and £32 000 raised from friends and patients will be an inspiration to others to take the plunge into the charity pool, for her legacy to the nation is helping patients with cancer every day.

1 Regents Wharf, 8 All Saints Street, London N1 9RL.

10 Signpost your hospital

J H Baron

Those who work in institutions know where they are and where they are going; they are rarely conscious of the notices and signposts. Doctors should, but alas do not, have more awareness of the problem of patients and visitors, all of whom, quite apart from their specific diagnostic fears, are frightened of the health care system in general and of hospitals in particular.

Patients and visitors have to make their way to a hospital and can be helped by a map being included in the literature sent out before admission. They need signs to tell them that they have arrived. They need to reach a particular part of the hospital and to know when they have achieved this objective. Each sign must be precisely located, of suitable size, material, and colour, and made up of legible and beautiful letters that suit the building.[1]

Anyone concerned with signposting a hospital must obtain a copy of *Signs*,[2] which provides full details of the Health Signs system and language. This chapter offers a personal user's guide for those who care about the visual environment of their hospital, whether old[3] or new,[4] and want to try to make their hospital both more efficient and more attractive.

Practicalities

The planner should pretend that he or she is, in turn, a driver, passenger, or pedestrian coming to the hospital, who needs to park, to reach a specific department, and from there other departments, and then to be able to find the lavatories, the cafeteria, and then the way out and back to the car park, all the necessary signs being still visible at dusk and by night.

Signs to the hospital

Those arriving at rail, underground, or bus stations need clear signs pointing towards the hospital, as from London Bridge station to Guy's. Those foolish enough to go to Hammersmith underground station hoping to find themselves near Hammersmith Hospital may need a kindly notice referring them to White City or East Acton stations instead. Car drivers need clear signs from town centres or major roads to the correct turn-offs. Many older hospitals are in back streets and they need signs from the nearest main road.

Proclaiming the hospital

Some public buildings can be arrogantly anonymous, like London clubs or Oxford and Cambridge colleges. A hospital should proclaim its name, be proud of its identity and its work, and assure visitors that they have come to the correct building.

Such declamation was taken for granted by the voluntary hospitals of the nineteenth century; the workhouse infirmaries skulked in shameful anonymity. Good Georgian examples in London included St George's, Hyde Park Corner (designed by Wilkin, 1827) and the General Lying-in Hospital, York Road (Harris, 1828). No one can mistake the Royal Waterloo Hospital for Children and Women (Nicholson, 1903–5) with its giant raised lettering in Doulton tiles.

The tradition continued into the 1930s in a variety of media. The old Westminster Hospital (Pearson, 1937) had raised metal letters on the façade to Horseferry Road, cut out metal letters lit internally at night over the main entrance, and letters incised in stone on the nurses' home. About that time came enamel on metal for smaller signs (for example, the Gordon Hospital). When the workhouse infirmary in Du Cane Road graduated into a teaching institution, an elegant sign of metal letters on stone arose and could be seen between the gates: HAMMERSMITH HOSPITAL AND POST GRADUATE SCHOOL OF LONDON; having lost a few letters over the years, there are now new signs.

The new Royal Free Hospital has preserved its 1894 semicircular cast iron sign from the old building, used classical raised metal letters for its school of medicine's façade, and used bold capitals mounted on a strip away from the main entrance wall to the new hospital. Neurologists (Maida Vale Hospital; Institute of Neurology) and psychiatrists (Tavistock Centre) stick to large plain capitals. But then came Health Service lettering (see below).

Finding the part that you want

Taxi drivers and some motorists need clear directions about where to drop passengers—be they patients or visitors—depending on whether they want accident and emergency, outpatients, or the main entrance for visitors. If departments are in independent buildings, it is even more important that outpatients, obstetrics, physiotherapy, and so on be signposted from the main road to the car parks nearest these units.

Car park notices, like all hospital notices, should not convey simply the usual warnings (CONSULTANTS ONLY), threats (YOUR WHEELS WILL BE CLAMPED), menaces (PENALTY £20), and disclaimers (BOARD OF GOVERNORS NOT RESPONSIBLE FOR LOSSES). Notices should be courteous and helpful: WELCOME TO ST CECILIA'S: PLEASE PARK HERE.

From the car parks, clear signs for the main entrance and inquiries should be placed so that no one, however anxious, could either fail to proceed in the desired direction or be left in limbo at an unmarked crossroads with alternative paths. Remember that many of your visitors have never been to your hospital before: do help them. Do not be tempted into the false economy of a small monochrome map surrounded and financed by local advertisements. Try for large maps showing, from the visitor's point of view and position ("You are here"), which buildings have which wards and departments on which floor, and by which staircase and lift they can be reached, with appropriate colour coding of the areas of different use. Designers specialising in axonometric drawings can construct these plans so that they differ only from the viewpoint of direction of approach. The alternatives are mere banks of signs, which can confuse by multiplicity unless they are grouped and broken down in the stages: AREA A ALL WARDS/OUTPATIENTS/ACCIDENT & EMERGENCY, as the visitor approaches a particular group. Try to be consistent: different signs in succession, such as ACCIDENT & EMERGENCY/CASUALTY/ EMERGENCIES, but all going to the same department are disorientating to the hapless patient.

Nor should the main entrance appear negative. Visitors are not charmed by their first impression of an NHS hospital: NO SMOKING/ SILENCE/NO CHILDREN UNDER 14. Why not WELCOME TO ST CECILIA'S, A

NO SMOKING HOSPITAL and PLEASE HELP US TO HELP OUR PATIENTS BY
TALKING QUIETLY?

Signs for wards, departments, and lifts

Although some of the older workhouse infirmaries still have wards
signified by letters and numbers, most hospitals new and old have
wards identified by a name, usually of a person, but occasionally of a
saint, street, or electoral ward. A personal touch is given to a ward
name if it is accompanied by a photograph or print of that person
together with a brief biographical note. The Royal Free Hospital has
a particularly successful set. Departments can be handled similarly
and named after former directors.

Detailed lists of the wards and departments on each level are
needed at the foot of staircases and in lifts, both beside each lift
button on each floor and inside the lift. It is helpful if when the lift
stops at each floor passengers see through the open gates a giant
number on the wall opposite denoting the level; similar indicators
are needed for those climbing stairs, whether main or emergency. As
you arrive on a floor you need signs for the direction and location of
each unit on that floor. Directions can be in identical format on each
level, but it is then helpful to have the floor you are at picked out in a
special colour.

Other signs

The tendency now is to number all doors. They also should have a
name, indicating the room's function or occupant, and the hospital
needs some central, identifiable, responsible, and dynamic person
who can order such name boards and, indeed, all other signs.
Nothing is worse than handwritten scraps of paper taped on to
doors, windows, or walls. Of course, temporary notes are needed;
they should be put neatly on prominent blank noticeboards. More
formal events boards with movable letters should list the timetable of
the day or week.

Manufacture

Signs cost money. A sign can cost £30–£40 to buy, and one sign
contractor quoted £120 000 for the initial phase of work on the site of
a hospital. The alternative today is "do it yourself". Sign writing
machines can be bought for about £25 000. Of course there will be
labour and material costs but at least you will be producing the signs
you want as and when required.

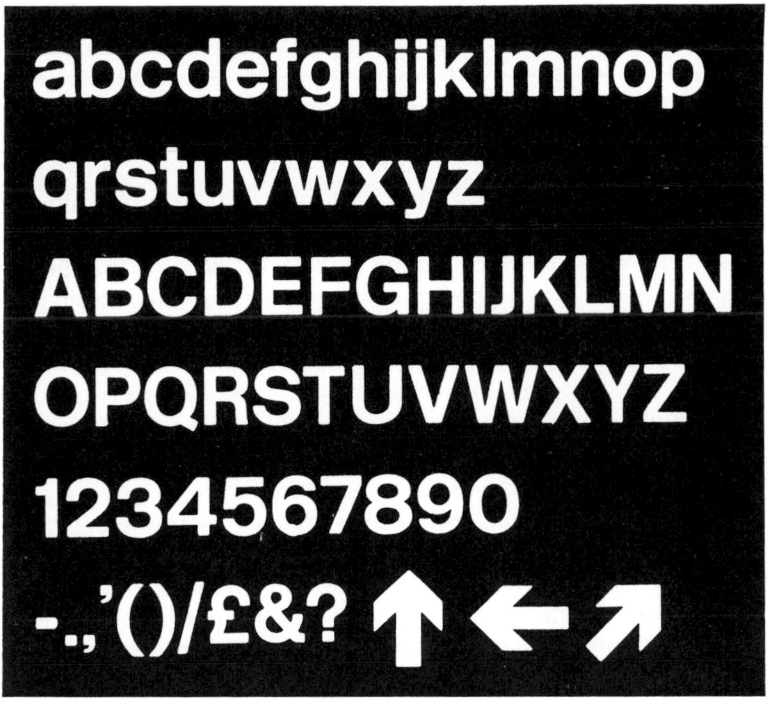

abcdefghijklmnop
qrstuvwxyz
ABCDEFGHIJKLMN
OPQRSTUVWXYZ
1234567890
-.,'()/£&? ↑ ← ↗

Fig 1 Health Alphabet

Maintenance

If your signs are washable or polishable, then someone must wash and polish them regularly; if they are painted, they will need painting often; and if they are separate letters fixed to a wall, they may go askew or fall off.

Battle of the styles—which lettering?

The NHS has a typeface all its own: the Health Alphabet (fig 1). It is widely assumed by health service architects, designers, and administrators, and even by doctors, that the Department of Health requires all hospitals to use this alphabet and no other when using the Health Signs language. This is a total misconception. The department indeed prefers hospitals to use Health Alphabet for economy, legibility, and a recognisable style, but *Signs* recognises individualism, and gives examples in Garamond, Clarendon, and

59

Rockwell. *Signs* rightly points out that, whatever style of lettering is chosen, there should be consistency of type for all the signs in a particular building and with the authority's coat of arms, symbol, and logo.

The early hospitals had lettering chosen, presumably by their architects, to be consistent with the style of the building. The former St George's is neoclassical, and the raised gilt lettering on the architrave of the portico is in a suitable neoclassical style, a formal announcement of classical monumentality in serifed letters. Most hospitals for the next 100 years retained a classical letter form. The alternative, a Roman letter without serifs, appeared on the Brighton Pavilion (1784) as English Egyptian type (1816), and as Grotesque ("Grot") in 1835.[5] With the beginning of the modern movement in architecture, design, and typography, the sanserif letter form was revived and has been widely used in the past 70 years, especially in Germany since the Bauhaus.

In 1915 Edward Johnston was commissioned by Frank Pick of London Transport to design the first standardised lettering for systematic use by a large organisation. The sanserif London Undergound typeface has survived successfully to this day. Johnston's pupil, Eric Gill, produced a sanserif type design of Gill Sans in 1927, which has developed into a family of different weights and widths. The medical world soon followed the trend, for example, in the London School of Hygiene and Tropical Medicine built in 1928 (Horder and Rees).[1]

The aesthetic problem of public lettering became acute when the Ministry of Transport's departmental committee on traffic signs reported in 1944 that "as legibility is important the standard lettering which we use for traffic signs is suitable for street names".[6] Local authorities were recommended to use a standard sanserif. Only rearguard action by letter lovers and the Royal Fine Art Commission persuaded the ministry to include in the recommended designs a serif alphabet, specially designed by David Kindersley in 1947.[6] When motorway lettering was to be standardised, however, Sir Colin Anderson's committee chose on aesthetic grounds Jock Kinneir's monoline sanserif upper and lower case (originally designed for the P & O and Orient lines, and later adapted for London Airport), rather than the Kindersley all-capital serif, in spite of the latter's being shown by the Road Research Laboratory to be more legible, even though the difference was not statistically significant.

Sanserif letters then strengthened their hold. In 1957 Max Miedinger had redesigned a Basle typefounder's Grotesque. Renamed Helvetica, it has had almost universal success since the early 1960s, not only as a typeface for printers, but also for signs, particularly since it became available as "Letrasign". In the late 1960s the Department of Health and Social Security commissioned Jock Kinneir to produce Health Alphabet, which is between a Helvetica light and Helvetica medium.[2] Health Alphabet, often called NHS lettering, has engulfed our hospitals old and new, just as when BEA and BOAC merged into British Airways in 1973 they chose for their new corporate identity a sanserif so as to seem informal, friendly, caring and non-pompous to the new young traveller.[6] Unfortunately, as Kinneir's Health Alphabet, Railway Alphabet and Airport Alphabet (designed by Fletcher, Forbes and Crosby) are so similar, their separate identities are lost. It is interesting that Colin Banks and John Miles gave the Post Office a totally different style of lettering in yellow on a red ground for its new image.[7]

Adrian Frutiger designed the signs for the Charles de Gaulle airport in Paris: his Roissy is a thin, elegant sanserif reminiscent of the Johnston Sans of 1915. When the new and fabulous MacKenzie Health Science Centre was built in Edmonton, Professor Bartl was asked to direct a project to design a sign system.[8] Studies on legibility led him to Frutiger 55 Roman (fig 2), which was therefore chosen throughout to "combine the advantages of modern sans-serif faces with the elegance and sensibility of classic type design".

But fashion in lettering, as in architecture and design, has now turned back again to the classical. At St Bartholomew's Hospital Anthony Williams, consultant in signposting to the Department of Health and Social Security used different alphabets (including a traditional serif type, Garamond), which are related in terms of colour, size, and proportion to the design of buildings of different periods. In 1983 I persuaded St Charles's Hospital to use Times New Roman (fig 3) throughout its 1881 buildings, and this lettering was also chosen for the new mental health buildings of 1985. Times New Roman was, of course, designed as a typeface for close viewing, with marked difference between thick and thin strokes, and is therefore not suitable for large buildings where notices are seen from afar. Both the British Museum and the National Gallery have recently redesigned all their signs, notices, and labels using letters with serifs: their designers, independently, and quite unknown to each other,

Occupational Therapy

External Psychiatric Services

Provincial Laboratory

Exit 114 Street

Cafeteria

Information Desk

X-Ray

Occupational Therapy

Emergency

Fig 2 Sample settings of Frutiger 55 Roman

ABCDEFGHIJKLMNOPQRSTUVWXYZ

abcdefghijklmnopqrstuvwxyz

123456789 ()!,.?;"

Fig 3 Times New Roman

chose Century Bold and Old, classical and monumental serifed typefaces (fig 4).

Doctors and scientists reading this account should by now be thinking of James Lind, and demand a controlled trial of legibility. Unfortunately, there have been few such studies in relation to signs, and the results conflict. When the laboratory evidence favoured serif, a committee still chose a sanserif upper and lower case for the motorway (see above). Several studies have rejected Helvetica and its related typefaces because they do not differentiate enough between individual letter forms to give optimum legibility of signs.

Other languages

Hospital managers automatically assume that notices should be in the English language in Latin script. Many parts of Britain have in their catchment areas ethnic groups with languages with non-Latin scripts—for example, Greek and Bengali. Expert advice should be taken to produce signs as beautiful and as legible as possible in these typefaces.

Campuses

Some hospital sites, especially at university hospitals, have two or more separate institutions on campus, and it is important to respect

ABCDEFGHIJKLMNOPQRSTUVWXYZ

abcdefghijklmnopqrstuvwxyz

123456789 ()!,.?;"

Fig 4 Century Bold

63

their individuality and autonomy. Thus at St Mary's where the hospital uses NHS lettering (soon to be replaced), I persuaded the medical school to use Times New Roman.

At the Hammersmith campus I persuaded the Arts Committee to set up a signs working party. A signage system has been developed to identify both the corporate personality of the site as a whole and the individual institutions. The lettering in the hospital is Century Old Style and identifies the hospital departments by ivory on maroon, the Royal Postgraduate Medical School by maroon on ivory, and the MRC Clinical Science by blue on ivory.

Conclusion

New hospitals must have a complete sign system, and most old hospitals will benefit from a revamping of the miscellaneous notices that have appeared over the decades. Remember, the system of signs is codified;[2] what you must decide is the type of letter. Basically, in the absence of good scientific field trials of legibility of signs, including their suitability for people with impaired vision, choices are still made on personal aesthetic grounds.

Certainly, use NHS lettering if you want to avoid controversy and save time, if you think it is the most beautiful available, and if you want your hospital to look like every other institution. If you want a modern sanserif, then there are several that are both legible and beautiful. If you prefer serifed letters, then you should look at old and new buildings that have them, until you find one you like that will suit your building. Then decide whether you want capitals or lower case letters. The choices are yours. Seize your opportunities—provided you are confident that you will not be upset by the inevitable criticism of your decisions.

Acknowledgements

I am grateful for helpful discussions or correspondence with Professor Peter Bartl (Edmonton), Peter Dormer (Ealing), Professor Fred Halter (Berne), Tony Noakes (DHSS), Professor Michael Twyman (Reading), John Weeks (London), Anthony Williams (Harpenden), Iden Wickings (London), Paul Wright (London). None of them is responsible for any of my opinions, errors, or conclusions.

1 Bartram A. *Lettering in architecture*. London: Lund Humphries, 1975.
2 Williams A, ed. *Signs*. DHSS Health Technical Memorandum 65. London: HMSO, 1984.
3 Baron J H. How to beautify your old hospital. *BMJ* 1984; **239:** 807–10.
4 Baron J H, Greene L. Art in hospitals. Funding works of art in new hospitals. Murals in London hospitals. *BMJ* 1984; **289:** 1731–7.
5 McLean R. *The Thames and Hudson manual of typography*. London: Thames and Hudson, 1980.
6 Crutchley B. *To be a printer*. London: Bodley Head, 1980.
7 Dormer P. *A closer look: lettering*. London: Crafts Council, 1983.
8 Bartl P. *Some pitfalls in signage systems for hospitals*. Icographic I/II Denmark: Mobilia Press, 1982.

11 Deal with colleagues with problems

David Roy, Jonathan Secker Walker

Relationships between medical practitioners, particularly in hospital practice, have always been complex, and attempts by colleagues or Trust Boards to intervene when problems arise often lead to much bitterness and ill feeling. We do not intend to go into great detail on the occasions when the law is concerned and the matter is dealt with directly by the disciplinary procedures of the General Medical Council (GMC), but to concentrate more on the difficulties encountered by doctors who are mentally ill, as well as those suffering from alcoholism and drug dependence, particularly when that illness directly affects the service that they are able to give to their patients. There will be discussion of the mechanisms existing to help doctors in such difficulties and a brief explanation of the current disciplinary codes for medical employees of the NHS.

Sick doctors

The medical practitioner's lot is traditionally perceived as a hard one, and few medical students enter their training without some idea, albeit minimal, of long hours on call, difficult life-or-death decision-making, and increasingly complex career choices with often dispiriting results. Many practitioners tend to be hard working, certainly ambitious, and to believe at the outset that they have resources to deal with an extraordinarily stressful way of life. In the past, however, medical schools have tended to play down this aspect of medical practice and so have colluded with the doctors they are training and the profession as a whole in propagating the myth that

66

good doctors subsume themselves totally to the practice of medicine with disregard for personal health and wellbeing. The emotional needs of doctors have, for the most part, been ignored, and medical students appear to receive little training in these crucial matters. It is not surprising that doctors in general have been slow to recognise the hazards of illness within the profession and the nature of these hazards, or that the methods of treatment and education deserve special consideration.

It is not easy to obtain data on the proportion of doctors who become mentally ill or develop alcoholism or drug dependence, and it seems that most surveys greatly underestimate the seriousness of the problem. Of doctors before the health committee of the GMC from 1981 to 1993, 86 were male and 12 female, and roughly equal numbers were in their 30s, 40s and 50s.[1] There were few cases in their 20s or 60s. The most common problem was mental illness (35/98), with alcohol (22/98) and drug dependence (14/98) the next commonest, and drugs plus alcohol accounting for 8/98. The split between general practice and hospital medicine was roughly equal. Many doctors seek treatment outside the official information-gathering services and it is possible that older doctors, who may be more liable to seek help for alcohol or drug dependence that has developed over some years, will be in a position to do so through the private sector. With the considerable increase in private health insurance this problem becomes more complicated, and the figures that are available from records of admission to NHS hospitals and referrals to confidential medical agencies must surely be the tip of the iceberg.

A major problem seems to be alcoholism, a paper in 1976 estimating there are 2000 to 3000 alcoholic doctors in the UK at any one time,[2] and, to a lesser extent, drug addiction, with a variety of affective disorders also being diagnosed. Schizophrenia and organic brain syndromes seem to be infrequent. An explanation for this may be that schizophrenic illnesses tend to present at a younger age, and may account for some drop outs from medical school, while organic brain syndromes would tend to predominate towards retirement. Certainly all the evidence suggests that rates of alcoholism, drug dependence, and affective disorders are noticeably higher in the medical profession than in the general population, as is the death rate from suicide and cirrhosis of the liver. The presentation of these syndromes is no different from that in the general population; alcoholic doctors have the same general medical sequalae and psychological problems as anyone else. The only difference may be that, given the doctors' medical training, they are more adept at hiding the problem from their colleagues and possibly, because of their perceived stigma in receiving psychiatric treatment, denying it to themselves as well. Marital disharmony may be an important contributing factor in the onset of mental disorder, or, indeed, may be provoked by it, and medicine is not renowned as the profession designed to keep marriages harmonious.

Alcohol and drug dependence

The available surveys indicate quite clearly that alcohol dependence is the major hazard among doctors. In a survey of 171 junior doctors in 1987, 4% described their alcohol use as heavy and frequent, and another 17% as heavy and occasional, while 7% used drugs for recreational purposes.[3] This is hardly surprising considering the high status that alcohol achieves as a drug in medical schools and as a social stimulant in later life together with the relative availability of marijuana and other soft drugs.

Given the increase in public awareness of problem drinking, the continuing campaign against drinking and driving, and the Royal College of Psychiatrists' report on individal alcohol consumption, which has resulted in a drastic lowering of the limit considered acceptable, there might be a reduction in these figures. Awareness of uninformed and uncontrolled alcohol consumption has, in the light of the alcohol policy formulated, resulted in the British Medical Association at one stage establishing a working party to investigate its own wine club.

Doctors who are drug addicts are as likely to suffer from personality disorders as an age-matched population of drug dependent people, and many medical addicts combine drug abuse and alcohol.

In a 1967 sample the list of drugs abused was headed by amphetamines and barbiturates, with heroin and methadone trailing. The pattern of drug use has changed considerably since then and with the dramatic reduction in the prescription of barbiturates, rarely prescribed nowadays, and the greater control of prescriptions for amphetamines, the tricyclic antidepressants and benzodiazepines acting as both hypnotics and anxiolytics are probably more abused. In the more serious cases that come to the attention of the GMC narcotic analgesic abuse is more common than abuse of other drugs.

Depression

In a review of psychiatric illness in British doctors in 1985, Rucinski and Cybulska generally concluded that the most common diagnoses remain affective disorders, accounting for between 21% and 64% of doctors' admissions to psychiatric hospitals.[4] Suicide rates for doctors confirm that depression is a relatively high risk factor[5]—especially in females.[6] Studies of junior doctors conclude that a larger proportion suffer from depression than the general population.[7,8]

The concept of "burn out" has gained currency in recent years. This syndrome can occur 10–15 years after practitioners are appointed to consultant posts and is often the result of waging the same battle over many years against a background of ever-tightening resources within the NHS, regular changes of senior managers, health service "reforms", complicated bureaucratic procedures, and an erosion of professional status. The rapid turnover of support staff, management structures that many clinicians feel undermine their areas of influence despite the introduction of directorates, and the large patient load, which is increasing in the face of diminishing resources and subject to the idiosyncrasies of the "market", often lead to feelings of isolation, helplessness, pessimism, and inertia. Occurring at a time of great vulnerability, this syndrome may also be partly explained by the concept of reaching a career plateau with nowhere else to go for the next 20 years.[9] After the numerous hurdles trainees must overcome to be appointed a consultant, the job at present is for life, without the need to continue to change, research or publish until retirement. It is still relatively unusual for a consultant to move jobs, except in academic medicine. This militates against those in high-pressure specialities like intensive care and neonatology being enabled to move sideways to less stressful arenas as they get older. Partly because of the frantic build up and race to be a consultant, subsequently to feel trapped or dissatisfied with the job may cause feelings of guilt in the individual, who, while surrounded by apparently contented colleagues, may believe the cause to be personal failure. It is not "the form" to explore these feelings with colleagues and the profession, and their teachers do little to prepare doctors for a problem that is probably quite common. Increasing lack of professional satisfaction may lead to demotivation, becoming "difficult" and irascible, and may account for some of the reasons for alcohol and drug dependence and depression.

Health education and the medical profession

It is clear that doctors face considerable and particular health problems, with attendant social and emotional consequences. Some medical schools have introduced counselling services for students, while others will deal with the more serious problems only when a student's performance is suffering. These necessary introductions are hardly innovative, and have lagged far behind the univesity campuses and colleges, where such services are an integral part of student life. This may highlight a problem in attitude on the part of the medical schools towards the emotional needs of their students, who will be the doctors of the future facing the appreciable health problems outlined in this chapter. Medical students should be encouraged to take part in counselling courses, which will not only teach a technique basic to the practice of medicine, but also enable students to engage in frank discussion of emotional issues. There is little discussion in schools of those aspects of medicine that do not appear in the textbooks, such as career choice and the increasing number of doctors failing to achieve their chosen discipline, management, relationships with colleagues and paramedical professions, being part of a team, and so on. Many of these issues will or should be part of specialist training in hospital, but the groundwork needs to be laid to avoid later problems. A straw poll among recent graduates from various medical schools indicates that they do not, on the whole, think that their medical schools deal with these issues satisfactorily, which is disappointing, particularly as pilot schemes have been introduced in some schools with success—although in others they have met with considerable resistance from the teaching staff and consultant body. The fact that most young graduates recognise the problem indicates that the schools are going some way towards facing it, and they should be wholeheartedly supported in this.

Problems in treatment

Doctors make bad patients. They find particular difficulty in accepting the role of patient, and there are certainly many professional tensions that arise between the doctor as patient and those who care for him, be they doctors, nurses, or others. The role of doctor as special patient further complicates an already difficult situation and may lead to early termination of psychiatric care on the part of the doctor. Although on one hand the therapist might be overindulgent or protective, on the other treatment given may be cursory because of the reluctance of the physicians to pursue the therapeutic options as vigorously as they would with non-medical patients, and this may result in poorer treatment and higher risk.

Mechanisms to help sick doctors

The "three wise men" procedure HC(82)13

Where information is received by the employer suggesting that a doctor may be suffering from physical or mental disability, including addiction, the chief executive, medical director, or director of public health may invoke the procedure recommended in HC(82)13, commonly referred to as the "three wise men" procedure. This usually works in an unobtrusive manner with a high level of confidentiality. Its status has not been tested in the courts, and it is advisory in nature. It is a precautionary and preventive measure, with the aim of heading off and treating disability in a doctor before a patient is harmed. It is non-disciplinary and seeks to lead to the doctor seeking a cure before disciplinary action is invoked. The medical staff committee of a hospital appoints three of their number who are respected and experienced to serve as the "wise" men or women for a set period. The organisation as a whole should know who they are, and feel able to approach them with concerns about individuals. Discreet soundings are taken initially and most cases lead to nothing except perhaps suitable advice to the doctor concerned. However, if the "wise" men or women feel that there is substance in the matter, a prima facie case will be presented to the doctor (in the presence of a chosen professional colleague if required), and if harm to patients cannot be excluded, the matter has to be taken further, often by the doctor agreeing to seek help from the National Counselling Service for Sick Doctors, described below. Refusal to follow the advice of the "wise" men or women may lead to a report to the GMC or to disciplinary action.

The National Counselling Service for Sick Doctors [10]

Machinery does exist within the NHS to regulate the activity of sick doctors whose work performance is causing concern, and the GMC has powers to inquire and intervene through its health committee. However, the National Counselling Service was set up as the result of an initiative by the president of the GMC and the

71

chairperson of council of the BMA in consultation with the royal colleges and their faculties. It is an autonomous organisation, which is controlled by a national management committee, and has appointed a number of national advisers, who are senior doctors representing all disciplines. After an informal contact by the doctor in need, or a colleague, the national adviser or a nominated specialist may contact the sick doctor, making an informal offer appropriate to his or her needs and outside the district in which he or she works. No records are kept at any central point, and should the doctor need continuing treatment, records will be kept only as a part of routine hospital administration This essential confidentality will, it is hoped, enable doctors to take up various offers of help. The Royal College of Psychiatrists has nominated 250 psychiatrists to act as counsellors in addition to 97 national advisers from various faculties. Anaesthetists may use the scheme described above, but also have a similar scheme for the speciality. Contact can be made through the Association of Anaesthetists.[11]

Sick doctors and the General Medical Council

Referrals through the National Counselling Service may fail or the situation may be too serious, and direct notification to the GMC may be needed. For many years the only mechanism of notification was a formal one, with a punitive referral to the GMC's disciplinary body. Since 1980 an informal confidential procedure exists whereby health authorities, trusts or professional colleagues (usually through the "three wise men") can initiate the screening of a potentially sick doctor by examiners appointed by the GMC. These medical examiners (two in each case) will report back to the preliminary screener on the doctor's fitness to practise. If it is then thought appropriate to impose certain conditions, such as the doctor accepting limitations on his or her practice while undergoing treatment, a medical supervisor, who may or may not be the doctor's treating physician, will keep the case under review, reporting back to the preliminary screener. Should satisfacory progress be made, no further action will be taken. Should these informal and fairly benign procedures break down, it would then be necessary for the case to be referred to the health committee, which may take statutory action by imposing conditions such as suspension. Only at this stage would notification of such a condition be passed to the employing trust hospital, community trust or family health service authority.

Issues of competence and problems of professional relationships

In addition to cases concerning sick doctors, problems of professional competence and conduct have caused major difficulties in the NHS, and there is considerable blurring of the issues in what can often become a *cause célèbre*, particularly where referral to the GMC is not appropriate. At the present time doctors and dentists, although subject to most of the disciplinary procedures of their employer, are treated differently from other staff groups in relation to the exercise of their profession while theft or physical violence, for example, would be treated in the same manner for all staff groups.

This is an area relating to the hospital's disciplinary procedures where the "three wise men" function may have failed to resolve a problem, or a particular colleague appears unable to relate to his or her peers, or have difficulties in running a department. Professional competence issues are probably more easily defined than those of professional conduct, the latter often being a symptom of some of the issues discussed previously. However, allegations of professional incompetence by other colleagues may be intimately related to clashes of personality and peculiar professonal behaviour. Clarity as to the real issues is essential before proceeding down a long and difficult path.

At present there is guidance from the Department of Health relating to issues of failing to honour contractual commitments, personal conduct, professional conduct and professional competence as well as the right to appeal against dismissal by the employer to the secretary of state (paragraph 190, *Terms and Conditions of Service*).

Disciplinary Procedures for Hospital and Community Medical and Dental Staff (HC(90)9) supersedes HM(61)112, which was originally circulated to health authorities in 1961 by the Ministry of Health. It updates the mechanism for dealing with serious disciplinary cases, introduces an intermediate procedure and professional review machinery, and alters the regulations for appeal under paragraph 190.

(1) Personal conduct is defined as "performance or behaviour of practitioners due to factors other than those associated with the exercise of medical or dental skills". In this case dismissal can no longer be followed by appeal under paragraph 190.

(2) Professional conduct is defined as "performance or behaviour arising from the exercise of medical or dental skills", while

professional competence is defined as "adequacy of performance of practitioners related to the exercise of their medical or dental skills and professional judgement". Both these types of misconduct can be dealt with under either Annex B, which is similar, but to a tighter timetable, to the process first described in the 1961 circular, or under the "intermediate procedure" Annex E, where dismissal is not felt likely to be the outcome.

(3) Professional review machinery is the appointment of a professional panel by a hospital to review the conduct of hospital consultants who are alleged to have failed to honour their contractual commitments.

The document relating to Annex B establishes a series of steps, starting from preliminary investigation for the establishment of a prima facie case and progressing through to a formal inquiry. These inquiries are formal and legalistic, requiring a high standard of proof, with many rights enshrined for the consultant under investigation, including the ability to comment on the proceedings, to make a plea of mitigation, and to appeal to the secretary of state. Although the revised circular set tight time limits for proceedings under Annex B, in practice they remain time consuming and lead to considerable cost to the various trusts or health authorities. There are currently several NHS consultants suspended on full pay pending such inquiries; each case may cost in the order of £250,000 and take inordinate amounts of senior staff time as well as subjecting the individual concerned to considerable stress.

The introduction of the less cumbersome Annex E, dealing with matters of professional conduct or competence that warrant disciplinary action sort of dismissal, was designed to speed up the process by appointing two independent professional assessors nominated by the Joint Consultants Committee from different hospitals to review the allegations, look at evidence, interview the consultant concerned and then recommend a course of action that stops short of dismissal to the employer. There is a limit of four months set for this procedure from the time the Joint Consultants Committee is asked to nominate the assessors. With the formation of NHS trust hospitals and units, existing consultants transferred with their current contracts and terms and conditions of service. Consultants newly appointed, however, have contracts that may be peculiar to an individual trust. Some trusts, while keeping to the broad outlines of the NHS terms and conditions have removed the right of appeal to the secretary of state under paragraph 190. At the present time it is not totally clear what will become of HC(90)9 as trusts employ an increasing proportion of their medical staff under individual contracts and different salaries.

Cases concerning professional conduct and competence in general practice will be directed to the family practitioner committee.

Conclusion

It seems that the procedure for dealing with a sick doctor has improved in recent years, although the reasons for doctor's greater vulnerability to particular health problems have received little attention. Support within hospitals for depressed clinicians is often meagre and the education of undergraduates and trainee doctors about the realities of practice could be improved. Where illness is not an issue, however, the relatively protected position of doctors is likely to change as NHS trust hospitals become increasingly autonomous. The current situation with regards to disciplinary procedures may look quite different in a few years time as the number of doctors on original NHS terms and conditions of service diminishes and individual NHS trust time-limited contracts become more numerous.

1 General Medical Council. *Annual Report.* London: GMC, 1993.
2 Glatt M M. Alcoholism: an occupational hazard for doctors. *Journal of Alcoholism* 1976; **11**: 85–91.
3 Firth-Cozens J. Stress, psychological problems, and clinical performance. In *Medical accidents.* Oxford: Oxford University Press, 1993.
4 Rucinski J, Cybulska E. Mentally ill doctors. *Br J Hosp Med* 1985; **33**: 90–4.
5 Steppacher R C, Mausner J S. Suicide in male and female physicians. *JAMA* 1974; **228**: 323–8.
6 Firth-Cozens J. Sources of stress in women junior house officers. *BMJ* 1990; **301**: 89–91.
7 Valko R J, Clayton P J. Depression in the internship. *Diseases of Nervous System* 1975; **36**: 26–9.
8 Reuben D B. Depressive symptoms in medical house officers: effects of level of training and work rotation *Arch Intern Med* 1985; **145**: 286 8.
9 Welsh E. Plateaus are boring. *BMJ* 1993; **307**: 944.
10 National Counselling Service for Sick Doctors, 1 Park Square West, London NW1 4LJ, telephone 0171-935 5982.
11 Association of Anaesthetists of Great Britain and Ireland, 9 Bedford Square, London WC1B 3RA, telephone 0171-631 1650.

12 Implement a no-smoking policy

Pamela Taylor

Implementing a no-smoking policy at work is all about successfully managing change. The steps to follow look deceptively simple on paper, so bear in mind it is people (employees) we are talking about and the need to change people's attitudes and behaviour at work.

An increasing number of organisations are introducing workplace no-smoking policies: some are pushed into it by their employees, some managements decide to initiate a policy, while others finally get around to rationalising a conflicting series of voluntary codes and obligatory regulations. In a major survey of employers almost 60% of respondents indicated smoking was their highest health promotion priority.[1] Most organisations have some form of restrictions on smoking somewhere on their premises. Mainframe computers have had the right to breathe smoke free air for over 20 years, staff handling food have been used to grabbing a quick puff in the toilets rather than in the kitchens, and nobody expects to smoke around a toxic chemicals area.

In the United Kingdom the majority of the population does not smoke and many people choose to avoid exposure to environmental tobacco smoke. The workplace is one of the last remaining areas where many non-smokers still cannot avoid others' tobacco smoke. Pressure from employees has certainly played its part in encouraging management to introduce policies, but some employers have taken the initiative themselves in an attempt to pre-empt any future legal requirements based on existing health and safety regulations, European Union regulations, and the law of negligence. The introduction of a well-planned no-smoking policy with careful consultation and presentation can be seen by employees as demonstrating management's commitment to the health, safety and welfare of its staff. Managing organisational change well has its spinoffs in improved internal communications and improved staff morale.

Voluntary codes?

It is pointless to raise the issue of smoking at work, risking antagonising employees, only to implement something which is clearly labelled "this code need not apply to you". Years of rows, arbitration, and management intervention await you based on continuing conflict and misunderstanding in the absence of a formal written policy. A voluntary code is no substitute for an agreed and properly implemented policy.

Reasons for introducing a policy

Health hazards

You will know of the health hazards associated with environmental tobacco smoke. Exposure causes eye irritation, headache, cough, sore throat, dizziness, and nausea. People with allergies and respiratory and heart ailments can also be seriously affected. Besides the acute effects of eye and throat irritation, exposure to tobacco smoke increases the risk of lung cancer and possibly of cardiovascular disease in non-smokers. As for the smokers themselves, about 81% of lung cancer deaths, 35% of all other cancers, and over 76% of cases of chronic bronchitis and emphysema are attributable to tobacco use, as are some 15–20% of deaths from coronary heart disease and stroke. The combined effect of smoking and occupational hazards shows there are significant differences in morbidity between smokers and non-smokers in many occupations and that the interaction of the two types of hazard increases the risk of many diseases.[2]

The law

Environmental tobacco smoke is a health hazard. Employers have a duty to protect the health of employees, and employees have a duty to protect the health of their work colleagues. Smoking in the workplace is a health and safety issue, and employers are required by statute law[3] (a) to protect their staff from workplace hazards and

77

(b) to keep abreast of new information on health hazards and to act accordingly.

There is a point at which a court will rule that the employer should know of new information and act—"the date of guilty knowledge". Some legal advisers believe we are at that stage now in view of the Froggatt report on the dangers of passive smoking. The report states: "The health risks to non-smokers of environmental tobacco smoke provide added argument for the overall reduction of smoking in the community, and non-smoking should be regarded as the norm in enclosed areas frequented by the public or employees, special provision being made for smokers, rather than vice-versa."[4]

Employers also have a common law duty to deal reasonably with matters of health or safety raised by their staff. So if you fail you could be sued for damages. A recent case saw an employee successfully claiming her asthma attacks were triggered by others' smoke.[5] The social security commissioner ruled this was an industrial injury case.

A good employer

Perhaps the best reason for introducing a policy is the desire to be a good employer, demonstrating your commitment to the health of all employees. Many trade unions have established specialist health and safety departments to look after their members' interests at work. The organisation Industrial Relations Services reports that unions play an active part in the formulation and implementation of workplace policies, particularly in the public sector, working with management.

Improve the ventilation and forget a policy?

Just in case you still harbour a secret desire to improve the ventilation system and forget the whole issue—it will not work. Both the particles and the gases in tobacco smoke contain irritants, toxins, and carcinogens. Some mechanical and electrical extractors can remove particles but they fail when it comes to the gases, which make up over 90% of the smoke.[6]

Taking it a step at a time

ASH (Action on Smoking and Health) runs a full-time advisory service to help companies introduce no-smoking policies. It recommends five steps: (1) setting up a working party; (2) informing the workforce; (3) consulting the workforce; (4) working towards a policy; (5) implementing the policy.[7]

Not another working party

Avoid the temptation to make do by extending the terms of reference of some existing working party. Smoking in the workplace is a big subject and it needs a specially constituted committee. By all means ensure your smoking policy working party has clear channels of communication with any relevant existing groups, but keep the working party separate, with its own terms of reference, directly accountable to the board or senior management body.

The size and composition will depend on the nature of the organisation, but give consideration to ensuring representation from management, personnel, industrial relations, unions or staff associations, or both, and staff representing office, shop floor, sales, and regional offices. You may wish to include some specialist health and safety, occupational health, and legal staff. Make sure both smokers and non-smokers are represented. Much time will be saved if the first meeting is used to ensure the objectives of the working group are clear. Make sure there is a written agenda and that agreed actions are written down.

The working party's role is crucial in striking the right balance between the gung-ho imposition of a policy and a talking shop that drags out the issue for months on end. An agreed outline timetable should be an aim for the first meeting together with agreed dates for future meetings.

Will a memo to all staff do?

The success or failure of your endeavour will depend on the working party's ability to communicate well, thereby creating an atmosphere receptive to change. A memo to all staff can form part of your communications exercise, but it is not sufficient on its own.

Check the usual channels of staff communication and use them. Implementing a no-smoking policy can often highlight poor employee communications in an organisation, so it may well be necessary to introduce some new ideas. You can consider health promotion programmes; it may be a good idea to distribute leaflets to all the staff on environmental tobacco smoke; posters can be displayed on notice boards; displays can be set up in canteens, sports areas, etc; articles can be written for in-house newsletters; or you may wish to bring in an outside expert to hold a series of staff briefing meetings. Once you have opened up the channels of communication with the staff, keep the information flowing. Make certain that your first efforts at communication with the staff include your aims to help smokers to quit. Most organisations set up special quit clinics during office hours and encourage their staff to attend. It is not unusual for these clinics to lead on to the provision of general stress control clinics for all staff.

I've informed them, so why consult them?

Informing staff of the health hazards of environmental tobacco smoke, employer and employee responsibilities on current legislation, and your wishes to implement a no-smoking policy all come before consulting the workforce. Now you are in a position to consult staff—which also ensures you act within the law. Consultation is a two-way process: resist any temptation to inform and then impose.

One of the most common methods of consultation is a staff questionnaire. A questionnaire helps gauge attitudes and encourages employees to think through the related issues. Some employees follow up questionnaires with one-to-one interviews, formal staff briefings, and follow-up questionnaires, which go into greater detail. The questionnaires can include questions on employees' opinions on whether smoking should be allowed at work and whether it should be restricted according to place or time; employees' own smoking habits and whether they would like to quit; whether other people's tobacco smoke bothers non-smokers, and if so in what way.

Other methods of consultation can include workplace ballots on suggested policy options, group discussions, suggestion boxes, computerised notice boards—anything that the working party believes best suits the culture of the organisation.

Policy? What policy?

Even if everything has gone well until now, deciding on the nature of the final policy can be harrowing. Is non-smoking to be the norm, with smoking breaks in designated rooms? Will you introduce a comprehensive no-smoking rule? The working party will need to gather all the relevant information to help reach a decision. What are the results of the workforce questionnaires? Is there an existing policy for some staff or areas? Where is smoking already banned to safeguard equipment or protect food? Could communal areas be a first step? Does practice vary from one site to another? Do you have to consider visitors or members? Are your offices mostly open plan? How are the smokers' quit clinics progressing? Bear in mind the key objectives agreed at the first working party meeting; remember the overriding need to protect non-smokers from tobacco smoke and to fulfil your obligations under health and safety legislation.

More and more organisations are opting for a comprehensive no-smoking rule on all premises. Some organisations opt for an interim policy of incorporating smoking breaks in designated rooms, making it clear they will progress to a comprehensive no-smoking rule after an agreed period. Others decide to review the policy after an agreed period without prejudice to the outcome.

Ready for action

Before you go live make sure the key players are fully informed on the policy the working party is proposing. Senior managers, union officials, and others must be satisfied they understand the policy, they appreciate how it was arrived at, they know how it will be implemented and monitored, and they are agreed on rules for compliance.

A survey of 100 companies showed warning periods of implementation ranging from two weeks to 14 months; the most common notice period was three months. There is a statutory obligation to consult under section 49 of the Employment Protection (Consolidation) Act 1978 and to give reasonable notice of any changes in employees' terms and conditions of service. Once staff have been consulted and the policy agreed it is necessary to implement it. Let the staff know the details of the policy and use the notice period as a further opportunity to communicate.

You could:

- update display materials on the effects of environmental tobacco smoke;
- produce a special staff newsletter and highlight the efforts of the staff who have managed to quit;
- commission specially designed posters and no-smoking signs to fit in with the organisation's corporate identity;
- replace any cigarette vending machines;
- place stubbing bins at entrances to smoking and non-smoking areas.

You could call a final meeting of the working party and ensure the

81

smooth handover to the personnel department. In particular, check responsibility for:

- handling the problems created by changes of staff accommodation,
- the monitoring of the policy,
- sorting out any initial problems with implementation,
- any non-compliance by staff,
- conditions and terms of employment,
- display materials and signs,
- progress with quit sessions for smokers,
- staff briefings,
- feedback on the running of the policy,
- monitoring the policy.

1 Smoking at work. 1—Why and how employers introduce smoking policies. *Industrial Relations Services Review and Report* 1992 Feb: No 506.
2 World Health Organisation Programme on Tobacco or Health. *Tobacco-free workplaces: safer and healthier.* Geneva: WHO, 1992. (Advisory kit.)
3 *Health and Safety at Work Act 1974* London: HMSO, 1974.
4 Independent and Scientific Committee on Smoking and Health. *Fourth report.* London: HMSO, 1988. (Chair: P Froggatt.)
5 Social Security Commissioner. Decision of the social security commissioner (re Joan Clay) appeal tribunal, 16 July 1990. Case No 2:11:1935.
6 United States Surgeon General. *The health consequences of involuntary smoking.* Rockville, Md: Department of Health and Human Services, 1986.
7 Jenkins M. *Smoking policies at work.* London: Health Education Authority, 1987.

13 Represent your colleagues

James Appleyard

Doctors' prime interest is the care of their patients. As this is both professionally rewarding and often very time consuming, it is not surprising that relatively few doctors have become sufficiently interested in the broad issues facing the profession to give time to representing their colleagues. For over a generation negotiations with the government over terms and conditions of service have continued centrally. The Doctors' and Dentists' Review Body has given an independent view about remuneration each year. The medical royal colleges individually and collectively in conjunction with the BMA at the joint consultant committee meetings have addressed major professional issues, including postgraduate training and staffing levels with the Department of Health. Universities are entrusted by the General Medical Council (GMC) with undergraduate medical education. The self-regulatory powers given in turn to the GMC by parliament under the supervision of the Privy Council have enabled professional standards to be maintained and any changes to occur at a pace the profession itself is able to adjust in the best interests of its patients.

Medical practice entails looking after individuals rather than groups. Doctors have traditionally worked independently in small practices in primary care or in small clinical "firms" or teams in hospital practice rather than collectively. This individuality and professional independence are the centre of our professional power, which arises from service to our patients. Like all power, if it is too tightly centralised it is much easier to take over and destroy. The present sharing of power and responsibility between the GMC,

BMA, the medical royal colleges, and the universities has maintained an important balance. None of the constituent groups has been able to seize total control of all aspects affecting the medical profession. All this is now changing.

Doctors have a deep sense of justice and fairness that is inherent in their everyday practice. Over the years they have tolerated a slow but inexorable erosion of their pay and status. Only when the pace of change becomes precipitate or when acts of gross unfairness are inflicted upon them do the members of the medical profession raise sufficient voices in unison.

The imposition of the NHS "reforms" was such an event—a major untried and ill-prepared structural alteration of health care provision into an unstable market system of purchasers and providers. This has been predicted by the computer-simulated "rubber windmill" game, played by some 40 experienced NHS professionals, to "crash" within three years! Responsibility for the service provision in the NHS has been delegated from the DoH to commissioning authorities. The Doctors' and Dentists' Review Body has clearly indicated that future pay negotiations will increasingly be conducted at local level.

Salaried doctors can no longer be protected by the "centre" and will not be allowed to continue their professional work on behalf of their patients without little direct managerial interference. This fundamental reorganisation means that there will need to be a much more robust local professional organisation to cope with professional and employment issues at local level. These changes have been anticipated by the BMA, which has set up a strong regional structure supporting the local negotiating committees accredited by it in NHS trusts. The current systems that safeguard general practice are likely to be affected by a similar process and many more doctors will be needed to represent colleagues locally in the future.

Few doctors in the past have set out on a medicopolitical career for its own sake. The issues are interesting—often far reaching—and the competition for key positions within the representative structure is at times challenging, but the rewards fall far short of those achieved through traditional clinical practice, particularly bearing in mind the enormous amount of unpaid work that is generated. At times of crisis the majority of doctors look to the small minority who represent them to "do something". Some of those seeking such action may get involved in the medicopolitical process and stay on. There are, however, some who seek office primarily to achieve wider political aims. As few doctors tend to vote for their colleagues in the "democratic" elections, the politically motivated can be sustained by a relatively small minority of support on narrow issues. The BMA has militated against "party political" domination of medical affairs, as inevitably the issues would then be seen more in national political than in professional terms.

Impatience, intolerance, and frustration with the democratic process breed pressure groups, which wax and wane according to the issues of the time unless they are propped up by wider political interests. Pressure groups have proved good training grounds for medical politicians. They command a disproportionate amount of power in relation to their numbers by the interest generated in the media. They make good copy in challenging the establishment and, because of their relatively small numbers, they are able to work as a closely knit team with limited but usually well-defined objectives. Challenging authority is one of the quickest ways of learning how the system works even if the system is thereby turned against you. Pressure groups rarely have the resources either in members or money to cover the great variety of medical, political, and professional activities and interests. They rapidly find they cannot impose their views on the reluctant majority, as there are limits at any particular time to what the profession will wear. Inevitably, to survive, the pressure group has to parasitise on the larger organisation with greater resources and access to better information. It takes time to change attitudes and often in this process, which requires a lot of patience, members of the pressure group get absorbed into the wider stream of BMA politics and adjust to the wider loyalties of the whole profession.

Knowledge of one's fellow doctors, knowledge of the current medicopolitical issues and knowledge of the system are the three pillars on which an effective representative must stand. How successful he or she will be depends on flair, ability, timing, and luck. There are some skills, however, that need to be acquired.

The general scene

Exciting scientific and technological advances have made rapid changes in medicine, and the public's expectation of what medicine in general and doctors in particular should achieve has risen. Progress in communication has made possible the widest dissemination of medical information, and patients rightly expect more time from doctors to discuss their problems and help them make their own decisions. Some of the NHS reforms encourage this process in principle, but in practice the contracting process has placed greater emphasis on money and overall numbers than on the individual needs of patients.

Doctors traditionally worked as independent professionals whose main source of income was their own patients. Third parties appeared when insurance schemes were introduced, and with the inception of the NHS in 1948 the medical scene was dominated by government as the main monopoly employer of doctors. General practitioners have fortunately retained some of their independence as independent contractors. The hospital and community health service doctors, who need more expensive support services, have essentially become full time employees. The interests of the two groups may conflict at times. The NHS reforms have been designed to divide up the profession and provoke conflict rather than cooperation. The NHS still has the monopoly of the market in health care but with a changing set of rules. Doctors have been caught up in this process both in the management structure as medical and clinical directors and in the medical staff and other advisory bodies. However, the ground rules change so rapidly. The new commissioning authorities have been seeking advice from a range of expensive management consultants and other professionals. Many of the traditional medical advisory structures have been allowed to wither. There is therefore a very urgent need to establish in each commissioning area a representative group from all medical disciplines that would be prepared to share a common vision for the local provision of services to patients. Such a group would need to monitor the performance of the commissioning authorities.

General Medical Council

The GMC has been given statutory powers to allow the profession a considerable amount of self-regulation. It is responsible for maintaining the standards of medical practice and for coordinating all stages of medical education: undergraduate, postgraduate, and continuing professional developments. Though half of the council is now elected, the traditional domination of the GMC by the university academics continues. With only a small proportion of the profession voting and a large number of candidates interested in gaining a place on the council, elections have proved an ideal

hunting ground for minority interests. Any doctors can put themselves forward in the quinquennial elections provided they are
supported by six of their colleagues. The BMA, on whose initiative
the GMC was founded in 1858, now sponsors some 22 candidates
and has gained more influence recently. There is to be a welcome
increase in the number of lay representatives on the council, who
play a very important part in the overall work. Recent consultations,
however, have revealed that the council will retain the support of the
profession only if it contains a majority of elected members. In turn,
it is important that these elected members reflect the wide spectrum
of views from within the profession.

Medical royal colleges

The medical royal colleges are responsible for the standards of
practice in their own specialties. They have become increasingly
responsive to the views of their fellows and members, and most of
their councils and committees are now elected bodies. The college
influence is still preserved on the advisory appointments committees
for new consultants and in their recognition of training posts in the
NHS. The colleges have embraced medical audit and are actively
involved in planning continuing medical education.

British Medical Association

The BMA is the political wing of the profession. It became a trade
union under the Trade Union and Labour Relations Act of 1974. It
is not affiliated to the Trades Union Congress (TUC) although it
does have informal contact with the TUC. The BMA is recognised
by the Department of Health and most local health authorities and
trusts as the sole negotiating body on behalf of doctors working in
the NHS.

The BMA is the recognised staff organisation representing the
medical profession on the General Whitley Council, on which the
staff side is composed of many unions, including Unison, the Royal
College of Nursing, and the Royal College of Midwives. In this
forum terms and conditions of service for all NHS staff have
traditionally been negotiated. By a special arrangement, the hospital
medical and dental services have been covered by agreements
reached in the General Whitley Council only if representatives of the
BMA's senior doctors (the Central Consultants and Specialists

Committee) and junior doctors, (the Junior Doctors Committee), and the Public Health and Community Staff (Central Committee for Public Health Medicine and Community Health) jointly agree that they should be. The senior and junior hospital staff join together to form a joint negotiating committee with the Department of Health, and doctors in public health medicine and community health have a separate negotiating board. General practitioners are independent contractors to the Family Health Service Authorities (FHSAs) in England and Wales, and to the Health Boards in Scotland and Northern Ireland. Each of the major committees within the BMA representing individual crafts has delegated responsibilities from the BMA council. Each has a regional structure to which local representatives are elected; in the case of general practitioners this is the local medical committee. Non-BMA members are entitled to join in these craft activities.

Local representatives

The parallel BMA structure exists through largely sleeping regional councils and the varying activities of the local BMA division. The BMA division nominates place of work accredited representatives (POWARs), who have been the professional equivalents of shop stewards. They must be BMA members. The POWAR may be the first point of contact with the BMA structure for doctors, and can refer problems to its full-time industrial relations officers and regional staff. Being a POWAR provides a useful introduction to the BMA organisation, with some real prospect of helping one's colleagues. Medical staff committees in each NHS Trust elect their representatives to a local negotiating committee. The majority of these are now accredited by the BMA and enjoy the experienced support of the BMA's industrial relations officers. Regional fora are held in order to inform and train their representatives. The BMA has a useful intelligence network nationwide. Consultation with the local staff organisations has not been a particularly high priority within the new "reformed" health service, but management should consult them over:

● strategic planning decisions, including the allocation of resources, which affect staff numbers and jobs;
● consequent administrative decisions, especially those likely to affect job prospects or job security of particular groups or occupations;

* all aspects of the work environment.

It is essential to have this local representative machinery in place to protect local doctors, who are increasingly vulnerable as individuals to the managerial machine. Each BMA division elects a representative to the annual representative meeting of the BMA. This forum is where the broad policies of the association are determined, which the BMA council, its executive body, is responsible for implementing.

There is thus a variety of different opportunities for doctors to represent their colleagues' views. Coordination and cross-representation ensures some communication between different parts of the medical system, but, as in any big organisation, this is still a real problem. The more active members become, the greater their need to be on several different committees so that the different activities can be linked.

Fellow doctors

Representation in the medical context is being a representative and not a delegate. There are no card votes in the BMA. Each representative is elected on his or her own merits and is entrusted to join in the discussions and debates on the various committees that have to make decisions. The local expressed view is borne in mind along with any new information learnt at the meeting. In contrast, a delegate has to vote according to the express wishes of the majority of the local group. If a representative clearly departs too far from the views of his or her fellow doctors, the democratic process within the BMA, which usually entails yearly elections, allows for his or her prompt replacement.

Doctors' contact with colleagues takes place largely in the course of their professional duties; sometimes informally over meals, at meetings at postgraduate centres, and on the different committees that we all have to attend from time to time, such as a hospital medical staff committee or the local medical committee. It is at these encounters that one can gauge the general feelings and attitudes of one's colleagues. When contentious issues arise, the discussion level or "grumble index" rises. If one becomes a representative on a national committee or advisory body, it is most important to listen to one's colleagues and keep in touch with the grass roots, or, as David Bolt, the former chairman of the Central Committee for Hospital

Medical Services, so aptly put it, with "what the profession would wear". In a brief spell as chairperson of the Hospital Junior Staff Committee and during my four years as chairperson of the negotiating subcommittee for consultants, I became all too aware of the potential isolation on such central negotiating bodies and of the important need for the appropriate feedback.

The strength of the BMA structure has relied on the fact that informed debate will occur at all levels, from the medical staff committee to the regional structure and the different subcommittees of the central groupings. Similar arguments and counter-arguments are raised and usually a consensus is reached. This may be a time-consuming process, but at least it ensures that professional representatives are in touch with the periphery. I once took a civil servant incognito for a hospital visit that included a canteen lunch at a district general hospital in the south east. Our companions at the table appeared at random, yet the conversation on the current issues was spontaneous and the same as we had been having centrally. This made quite an impression on the civil servant, who admitted he had never actually visited a hospital before. We won our points!

Current issues

A glance at the agenda of different committees within the BMA or the medical royal colleges will show the same problems recurring year after year. On many of the issues there is a balance of opinion, and in the cycle of time one or other of two opposite opinions predominates. Any action sets in motion the process of reaction. This has been most noticeable during the past 20 years on the intractable problem of how to resolve the imbalance of medical staffing levels. This has been an issue that has started many a young doctor on a political career. It seems so simple, just a matter of numbers, until you realise that there are a lot of different factors involved and that with each the equation becomes increasingly complex. The pursuit of one "simple" solution can cause serious disruption in the provision of medical care. The main influence on staffing levels is, of course, financial.

The NHS embraced the profession, and the profession, in turn, has become so involved in the NHS that the whole concept of the health service free at the time of use is now part of our medicopolitical culture. Doctors have become proud and protective of the service, and they invest an inordinate amount of good will by working far in excess of their strict contractual duties in order to make it function. Doctors have been critical too, continually asking for more money and for better facilities for their patients. Their terms and conditions of service have specifically allowed practitioners the freedom, without prior consent of the employing authority, to publish books, articles, etc, and to deliver any lecture or speech whether on matters arising out of their hospital service or not. In the new system many modern managers find this paragraph difficult to come to terms with. Doctors are becoming increasingly under pressure not to reveal the embarrassing information about the inadequacies of the health service. Individually they are extremely vulnerable, and it is only through the support available in the BMA that management can be challenged. The good will of the medical profession has been a major feature of the NHS. The continuing commitment of consultants has traditionally allowed growth and stability to occur from a stable base, but the present contracting system has introduced a major element of uncertainty. Contracts can be changed at the whim of management with or without a token medical consultation. This instability, combined with the traditional drive and good will that doctors have been giving to the health service, has promoted conflict and confusion. The preservation of the traditional values of the medical profession of service to patients is increasingly important. Even in times of great dispute the profession has always shrunk from exercising the right of strike action. It is always important when disputes occur to remember that it is the government that has the responsibility of deciding on the level of health care that is provided, but that doctors have the duty to care for their patients irrespective of whether they are seen in or outside of the health service. Resignation from the NHS is the ultimate weapon. A strike against patients will lead to the ultimate demise of doctors as professionals.

Ethical issues related to medical practice have been major topics of discussion within the profession. There have been some excellent debates at the BMA's annual representative meetings. In general, the public respects doctors' opinions on medical subjects but the further away from the practice of medicine the topics discussed are, the less respect is given to any pronouncements by the BMA. There is always a serious danger of alienating patients and devaluing medical opinion when doctors express contentious sentiments about social issues that are the particular concern of the general body politic rather than any specific professional group.

Skills

The main assets the representative needs are time, patience, and tenacity. Medical issues generally take some time to resolve. Events, however, may move fast, and that is when experience and wise judgments are needed. It is important to remember that you never get owt for nowt. Some important skills are needed in committee work and negotiation, and recognising this, the BMA offers appropriate training. Such courses provide important and interesting insight into one's own abilities, strengths, and weaknesses, and, if nothing else, can reduce the number of mistakes you make, thereby ensuring better results in negotiation. These skills can be broadly classified as proper planning and appropriate behaviour. First, it is important to find out as much information as possible about a particular topic and decide what the particular issues are. After this, you need to canvass opinion and build a professional power base by getting support for your objectives from as wide a section of the profession as possible. Then you need to understand the various political forces at play on the particular problem you are facing in order to set ultimate objectives and achievable targets, as well as consider a "fall-back" position and the "bottom line".

In dealing with other people the professional training required by a doctor comes in useful. It is important to listen to the various arguments and to hear what others are saying. One must be able to work as a member of a team in any negotiations, with some members doing the talking and others doing the listening. Tension can mount and in these circumstances it is usually those who keep their cool that win in the end.

After such negotiations on behalf of colleagues it is very important to debrief, to review the proceedings to see what has or has not been achieved. It is essential to keep colleagues fully informed about the progress of any discussions. It is the hallmark of a good representative to share ideas and information with those he or she represents so that they, in turn, can make informed judgments and their views be properly represented.

Is it all worthwhile?

With the knowledge and support of colleagues our representatives can make progress in improving patient care and defending the independence of the profession, on which the individuality of each patient depends. The price of freedom is eternal vigilance. It is up to us to become involved through the local representative machinery and ensure that our representatives are alert to the changing circumstances. If you are unhappy about your own representative's performance and have the time, toughness, and tenacity, why not try yourself?

14 Organise your time

Douglas Black

It is lucky for writers of didactic articles, and perhaps also for doctors in general, that we are not rigidly constrained to practise what we preach. For this particular subject I have the uneasy feeling that I must have wasted a good deal of that precious and limited commodity, in excess of what I have been successful in organising. But there are two pleas to be made in mitigation: the possessive pronoun in the title is "your" and not "my"; and I have had the salutary experience of working for and with people who by any standards would be considered to have used their time wisely. So let me try to tell you what I have learnt from them while still making no claim to have emulated them.

A time for every purpose

Perhaps the first thing to recognise is that the greater part of time for most of us is not open to be organised. We are not, of course, any longer constrained by the old agricultural adage "Eight hours to work, eight hours to play, eight hours to sleep"—and still less by its tailpiece, "and eight bob a day". But all of us need some sleep, whatever the variation in requirement between individuals. And the balance of opinion is certainly in favour of some equivalent of "play", not discounting, however, those fortunate enough to find their recreation in their work. "Dulce est desipere in loco"*—and I

---

* For, when the time and place are right
  'Tis sweet to make good cheer.—HORACE (translated by Lord Dunsaney)

remember from some years back how a rather tedious faculty discussion on what could be permitted, or not permitted, in an elective period was brought to life by the suggestion from our enlightened dean, Colin Campbell, that provision ought to be left for the young man who just wanted to lie in a grassy field and think. But even if we stick to that part of time designated as "work", for most people in most occupations it tends to be organised for them rather than by them. We doctors are more fortunate than most, but it is the rare freelance among us who is not to some extent the creature of the system.

I hope that in saying this I am recognising a fact of life, and not disparaging routine, which is something that we all need. Indeed, it can be wonderfully comforting during the periods when some apparently more creative activity seems to be going badly; I recall how in the days when I did research and things were going badly it was a considerable solace to undertake either a teaching session or an outpatient clinic. But such activities, however comforting and in their own way challenging, are normally dictated by timetable and not by personal initiative and organisation.

Even after making all these deductions for sleep, recreation, and routine, there still remains for most of us some time that we think we can organise. Before I turn to specific aspects of organising time for particular tasks, there is one piece of general advice which could be summarised thus, "Discover your own tempo and work with the grain of it and not against it". I have already mentioned that we need differing amounts of sleep; and it is better to be awake during an examination than to have spent a wakeful night before it in what may be a panic effort at catching up. But we also seem to need sleep at different times of the 24-hour cycle. We may not discover this in the set routine of our schooldays, but in the comparative freedom of the university we soon discover whether we are larks or owls. It is sensible to recognise which we are, and to concentrate as far as possible our most original tasks in our best time of the day. I learnt from Leslie Witts that this is not the same thing as being idle when not at one's best; he was fond of quoting from Matthew Arnold, ". . . tasks in hours of insight will'd/Can be through hours of gloom fulfill'd".

Another general principle is perhaps to try to devote as much as possible of your disposable time to things that you are good at. The difficulty here, of course, is to discover what these things are. The hedonist in me says, "If you are enjoying doing something, you may

95

be doing it well", but the puritan in me says, "That may be a necessary criterion, but it's not a sufficient one—you may be enjoying it, and still doing it jolly badly". Self assessment also has the weakness of wishful thinking—I have known superb clinicians who misdiagnosed themselves as researchers, and conversely. It is not always easy for young people to recognise the direction of their own talents, and it may be the duty of a tutor or the head of a department to help here, difficult though advice of this kind may be to give or to take. Of course, with the passage of time more objective evidence may appear—clinical success brings patients, academic success increases the ratio of accepted to rejected papers and communications to societies. I am not, I hope, suggesting that we should attempt only those doors that yield at a touch; but if repeated attempts suggest that they may be locked, it might be an idea to try something else. And, of course, on a longer time scale, the things that you are good or bad at when you are young may not stay that way throughout life—even quite foolish people may learn from the rigours of experience.

Academic questions

Coming to more specific matters, as an academic I had to apportion my time among clinical work, research, teaching, and administration. As the more inescapable components, clinical work and teaching run fairly constantly through an academic career; but as time goes on it takes more resolution than I possess to prevent administration from encroaching on the time available for research. For many of us, election to a chair marks the transition from personal to vicarious research, as was crystallised by George Pickering when he told me, "Your job now is to enable other people to do research". Sadly, this must be a task of increasing difficulty for today's professors, but it remains a very important part of their responsibility. Discussing their research projects with younger colleagues, and helping them to present their results, is a first call on the time of a professor. Organising time for personal research is very much an individual matter—for some it is an all-embracing priority, for others it fluctuates with other interests, and also, let us face it, with how well the research is going. And again, teaching is largely a matter of timetabling and opportunity, not greatly susceptible to personal organisation. May I then devote the rest of this chapter to some aspects of the organisation of time spent in clinical work and in administration.

Patients included

The times of ward rounds and of outpatient sessions are usually part of an established hospital framework but the way in which the time so allotted is spent leaves much to individual initiative. What I know of the essentials of clinical organisation I owe to the experience of working for over 20 years with Robert Platt, who taught me that everything must be centred on the patient at the bedside, technical discussion of the illness being reserved for the second half of the round, perhaps over tea. Similarly, in a clinical meeting the worst crime in his eyes was to present a case history without bringing the patient into the conversation.

In the outpatient clinic, working independently, I had, of course, to make my own discoveries on the use of time—for example, that a teaching clinic, as James Spence emphasised, is an opportunity for one or two students to witness the process of a consultation, not an occasion for giving mini lectures or answering questions on the nature of disease. I learnt that if the day's work is to be done in the day a history must be guided, and not left to free association. More painfully, I occasionally suffered from being at the receiving end of someone else's organisation of their time at my expense. This is perhaps a cryptic way of describing the situation in which a patient from another hospital staggers into the room laden with 20 pages of notes, a bundle of x ray films, numerous investigations on unfamiliar forms—everything but a summary and a statement of the problem. On such occasions one has to take a deep breath, explain to patients that there is a lot to look through, apologise for keeping them waiting, and generally do one's best, conscious that patients are likely to have had their expectations raised by whoever referred them. Managerial and sociological advocates of tight appointments systems, please note.

Committee insomnia

As in clinical work, in administration much would seem to be predetermined—the times of boards, committees, examinations, and so on. But individual flexibility creeps in when we consider the way in which the time is actually spent. Because of their critical importance to individuals, I believe that examinations and appointments committees demand the entire concentration of all concerned, and I would be a little worried if an examiner did not feel spent at the end of a day of clinicals and orals. But in most other committees it would be flattering to describe the proceedings as of uniformly high interest. I have never quite had the hardihood to imitate those of my colleagues who visibly get ahead with their correspondence during meetings. I also believe that it is desirable to stay awake, even if arousal is maintained by interest in the people rather than in the business. There is always, too, the possibility that out of a cloudless sky there may come a sudden storm, threatening the body whose interests you are there to represent.

Many years ago I described a syndrome from which I myself suffer: committee insomnia. I have not yet found a cure, but for those who suffer from its opposite (inability to stay awake in committees), I recommend becoming chairperson. In that event, however, it is wise to spend a little time beforehand in considering the course that the meeting is likely to take. For major meetings at least, the civil service has a briefing meeting beforehand and a debriefing meeting afterwards; given a competent secretariat, such an array of procedures does more for full employment than for an economical use of collective time.

Seizing the day

Finally, are there ways of "saving time"? Perhaps there are, though it is not easy to prove. Time can certainly be lost by frequent interruptions and by lack of concentration—so you can make use of train journeys and plane journeys and, more riskily, of car journeys along familiar daily routes. Time spent in sleep may not be wasted, even intellectually—nocturnal solutions of a problem have been described. I have sometimes noticed that unusually clear formulations come to mind on first waking—and not all of them are transient, even if they mostly fade into the light of common day.

15 Set up a patient participation group

Tim Paine
Revised by B E Marks

Patient participation is emerging from its infancy as a new enterprise in general practice. It has become an increasingly common topic for discussion and debate at meetings and conferences, and the number of practices with a patient participation group (PPG) is steadily rising. Although there is still considerable resistance to the idea, especially among long established general practitioners, the number of doctors seriously considering it has multiplied. The principle behind it is as old as the hills: the best results occur when client and craftsman confer over the job to be done and pool their resources in carrying it out. This is the basis of counselling, and patient participation is simply counselling writ large. A PPG is not, and should not be, the only means of participation. Every consultation is an opportunity for sharing—information, insights, solutions, and tasks; a PPG is merely a structured and practical method of consultation with the practice as a whole.

What is a PPG? There is enormous variety among the 120 or so in existence, but most share a basic structure. A committee of patients (who may be elected by their peers, or co-opted), together with one of the partners and one or more of the practice team, meet at regular intervals to decide ways and means of making a positive contribution to the services and facilities offered by the practice to its patients. Patient participation group activities tend to fall into five main areas: consumer feedback—a voice in practice planning and organisation; health promotion—meetings, group literature; community care— various voluntary activities such as transport, fetching prescriptions, and social events; providing information—practice guides, leaflets, local facilities; and fund raising—both to maintain the group and to purchase equipment and provide facilities. By no means all groups engage in all these activities; some prefer to limit their energies to one or two. It very much depends on the interests, priorities, and talents of those concerned and how much time they have to spare.

What have practices gained from having a PPG? For many who have become involved—patients and professionals—it is the atmosphere of openness and mutual respect that seems to go with participation that is the most important plus. Others will point to more tangible results, such as a woman partner, a better organised appointments system, or a more congenial waiting room—the results of feedback and suggestions. A health education programme, patient transport service, or lunch club for the elderly are further examples; the list is long. Arguments for having a PPG range from the basically practical (more involvement: better system), to the philosophical (freedom and autonomy) and the political (public service: public say).

Selling the idea

The first task that anybody thinking of starting a PPG should attend to is reading up on the subject. The superb little book by Ann Richardson and Caroline Bray called *Promoting Health through Participation* is now out of print, but may be available in a library, and is still a useful mine of information for anyone about to take the plunge. It is also a valuable guide to publications about patient participation.

If you are inspired by what you have heard and read, and want to proceed, the next step is consultation—with partners, team, and maybe one or two "likely" patients. A large part of this is a selling exercise, and it may tax your powers of persuasion to the full. It is to equip you for this that background reading and thinking are so vital, so that you are sure of your facts and arguments. Of course, the other object of the exercise is to listen to people's reactions and suggestions; "bulldozing" will get you nowhere. One of the reasons groups fail (and this happens not infrequently) is that those concerned have not talked things through sufficiently before they start. This may lead to unrealistic and conflicting expectations, and eventual disillusionment. Do your best to encourage active participation from the start. This applies especially to the practice team and staff, who are all too often left out of discussions and plans, and not surprisingly show little interest subsequently. Receptionists and health visitors in particular are valuable allies in the initiation and running of a PPG, and the more opportunity they are given from the start to contribute ideas, suggestions, and their time to the scheme, the better will be the prognosis for the group. To make it easier for everyone to gain a clear impression of what a PPG implies, consider inviting one or more people from a thriving group to meet your practice and talk about their experiences.

The National Association for Patient Participation (NAPP) represents practice patients' groups nationally and receives support from the Department of Health, which is sympathetic to its attitudes and aspirations. Its main roles are to encourage the formation of new groups, help with the activities of established ones, and act as a resource and point of contact for individuals and organisations interested in patient participation in general practice. Each year NAPP holds a national conference on health issues of particular concern to patients' groups, at different venues throughout the country, often attended by its patron, Lady Chalker.

NAPP's secretary (Mrs Ann Smith, 11 Hardie Avenue, Moreton, Wirrall L46 6BJ) will on request send a "start-up" pack, together with the name and address of the regional officer responsible for the area. The role of the regional officer is to aid the work of local groups and to arrange regional meetings at which groups get acquainted and share ideas and experiences.

Once the preliminary discussions are under way, it won't be long before you know if you are on to a winner. It is probably wise to satisfy a few basic criteria before proceeding further; an enthusiastic doctor willing to devote several hours a month, at least initially, to establishing and supporting the group—that's you; partners who are well disposed to the scheme—or at least not antagonistic; one or two members of the practice team who are willing to help enthusiastically; and possibly one or two patients willing to act as catalysts for the first year or two. (You may, of course, decide to delay the involvement of any patients until you are ready for the launch.) Having obtained general agreement, you will need to form a small planning group to examine logistics in detail. Perhaps the more vital aspect to consider is the operational philosophy of the PPG. If you and fellow planners have democracy and accountability at the top of your list of priorities, you will probably opt for a committee elected by the practice list and totally autonomous in deciding the range of its activities—so you may decide merely to float the idea at a

101

meeting, describe a few PPG activities and benefits, and let them get on with it. On the other hand, you may want to be a little more directive (in the interests, of course, of PPG effectiveness), and present interested patients with a structure for the group, a list of initial activities and even a constitution. If you veer towards this stance, you will need to work out some practical details about how such activities as feedback, health education, and community care might be organised and put into operation.

Funding and publicity can both pose problems. Unless they become very elaborate, PPGs are relatively inexpensive to set up and run. Most groups manage on less than £500 a year, and probably need only £50–100 to get started. Partnerships often contribute this sort of money at the start, and annually thereafter, which is, of course, tax allowable. It is well worth approaching health authorities, particularly if the group is to have a health education role; and local firms and charities are other sources of funds. Once the group is established, it may well become self financing from fundraising activities such as jumble sales, raffles, and sponsored events.

Publicity is probably the biggest headache that you and the group will have to cope with. The constraints on professional advertising are in the process of some degree of relaxation, but it is unlikely that practices will be able to publicise PPG activities other than directly to their own patients. (The one exception is a health education event, which may be widely advertised as long as the practice itself is not identified.) As you will probably be aiming for a maximal response from your patients at the start—most PPGs begin with an open meeting to discuss the scheme—it is worth making a supreme effort to reach as many on the list as possible. This means giving serious consideration to supplementing publicity at the surgery or health centre with a distribution of letters to homes, even through the post. It is also worth putting a lot of thought into how you present your message. The wording and visual impact are crucial, and your planning group may decide that it is helpful to seek some expert advice. Experience has shown that patients respond most positively to communications directly from their doctors, so arrange for the whole partnership to sign the letter before it is duplicated.

When the planning group has done its work, it is wise to have a final practice meeting before the launch, with the proposals and details down on paper. From this stage on it is a good idea to minute discussions and decisions, if only to prevent individuals having an excuse for claiming that they were kept in the dark.

Carrying it through

By this time you and your fellow planners are likely to be somewhat excited and impatient for the huge response to the publicity that you have so carefully engineered. A note of sober caution must be sounded at this point: patient participation is not everyone's cup of tea, and this applies to patients as well as doctors, so don't be too downcast if only 10 or 20 people turn up to hear more about it. Lots of successful groups have started very modestly. If you have opted for a meeting to promote the scheme (some practices start an activity first, such as a community care scheme, and develop a PPG from there), your presentation and selling skills will again be needed. Try to give everyone who comes a chance to feel involved from the word go. Breaking the meeting up into groups of six or eight to discuss among themselves what you have just told them (there's no need to move into separate rooms) will get people thinking and enthusiastic. Something that appeals to a lot of people is to feel that they are being given an opportunity to contribute to a worthwhile experiment; there's also a strong tendency to want to make an experiment work. Before the meeting breaks up, you will need to ask for volunteers for the steering committee. Most groups have about 12 patients on their committees, but this may be too many to aim for at the start, Too much arm twisting is usually self-defeating in the end, so start small and build up. If you have already found one or two patients who are willing to act as a committee nucleus, it will make things that much easier. The numbers who volunteer will to a large extent determine the range of activities of the group. Avoid being overambitious; people, including you, will be put off by the number of jobs they have to do. There is, however, an advantage in having a selection of PPG activities. If any prove unsuccessful, the group has other eggs in its basket.

There is often some doubt as to how closely involved the doctor(s) should be in the operation of a PPG once it has commenced activities. My own experience may be relevant. I announced that, having come up with the idea, I now thought that running of the group was up to the patients. I felt it was wrong for a doctor to be influencing a scheme set up to give the patients a voice of their own. It wasn't long before the steering committee began to resent my apparent distance from the group, and the lesson I learnt was that you cannot have one-sided participation. The compromise, which seems to have worked, was for me, or one of my partners, to attend committee meetings by invitation, and as many of the group's evening meetings as possible. Visible support from doctors goes a long way to maintain PPG morale.

The first year or 18 months of a PPG's life is usually straight-forward. Troublemaking patients on the committee are seldom a problem; but if they are, their fellow members usually sort them out and they go away without a receptive audience. (I don't mean by this that groups should avoid all criticism of the way the practice is run. Constructive criticism, and coming up with alternative solutions to problems, is part of their *raison d'être*.) Once the novelty has worn off to some extent, and the founding members start to feel they have done their bit, a period of doldrums and doubt can overtake a group. New blood is needed, and everyone wonders where it is going to come from. This is a time to inject some extra special effort again. It may be worth carrying out an honest review of the group's achievements and likely potential, and, if everyone agrees it is right to continue, to organise another big publicity drive. Once a group is over this phase of post-honeymoon blues, momentum tends to be maintained. One of NAPP's assets is the opportunity it provides for PPGs in different regions of Britain to meet each other and share experiences. It is a great boost to a struggling group's morale to hear that other people have had similar problems, and have found ways of solving them. One of the commonest frustrations is the unwilling-ness of patients to participate. You have to recognise that it is a minority interest—probably attracting the same proportion of peo-ple in a community who might want to attend evening classes. So to achieve a satisfactory response to any meeting, say, one has to make the subject sound relevant to the audience in question, and this again is where skills in communication and "selling" are so valuable.

Setting up a PPG is challenging and exciting, and not without certain risks. One of the refreshing things about PPGs is the lack of standardisation; every practice, and every group, must do its own thing. I have merely suggested a framework, and I am sure no one will feel bound to stick to it. Have a go . . . and good luck.

16 Cope in office

Tom Solomon

"How on earth did you cope with it all?" asked my successor, as I handed over the reins of office. Twelve months previously, when I had started as president of Osler House Club, Oxford's Medical Student Union, I had been similarly daunted. Of course all the relevant files had been passed on to me, but I soon realised that there was so much more to it than that. Even a flick through the previous editions of these books, helpful though they were, did not teach me some of the basics that seem vital for someone taking on this sort of responsibility for the first time. Much of what I have learnt will, I am sure, prove to be of value to the many medical students and junior doctors who will find themselves in increasingly managerial roles in the future.

Time management

Whatever the particular management role you have taken on, it will soon become apparent that your own degree of organisation will make a big difference in determining how well you cope. Crucial to this is how effectively you manage your time. However plush your Filofax, there will still never be enough hours in the day for everything you would like to do. But one way in which you can ease this difficulty is by limiting the constant interruptions that seem to be part of the job. Initially, you like to feel that you are always available for people to pop in, "My door is always open," you say. But you will soon realise how much of a time waster this can be, for not only is there the delay while you talk to your visitor but there is

105

the additional inefficiency of having to keep stopping and starting. Far better to set aside a period—perhaps five till six every evening in the bar—when people know that they can catch you. Similarly, though being offered a hospital bleep may be a tremendous boost to the ego of an aspiring medical student, the scope it allows for unnecessary interruptions means that you are far better off without it. You can be too readily available for your own good.

Never ending post, though initially flattering, soon becomes a source of headache. At first I tended to open the day's post in a spare five minutes, just to see if any of it appealed, then I would look at it again later. Over the next few days some letters would be read a third or fourth time as I answered them. Others would lurk at the bottom of my bag for weeks before I would finally get around to answering them or throwing them away. This rereading of the correspondence was obviously highly inefficient. In a mood of ruthless efficiency I developed a "handle it once" policy. The post would remain untouched in my pigeonhole until I had sufficient time to deal with it all in one go. If this meant I had to ignore it for a day or two, then so be it. Once opened, however, it would be answered straight away so that each letter would be handled just once and dealt with there and then.

Replying to letters is also a potential time waster if you are not careful. It amuses me to see how my successor—just as I did at first—diligently types out beautiful replies for all his correspondence, however trivial or unimportant it may be. You soon learn that for most of it a reply scrawled on notepaper or even across the bottom of the received letter will do. Why waste half an hour carefully explaining to Hackmann Stethoscopes that you do not think students will be interested in a "special £1 reduction" offer on the new cardiology scope, when a simple "not interested, thank you" will suffice.

Committee life

To ensure smooth running of committee meetings a great deal of tact and skill is needed. It is worth first considering how the meetings will work. Will someone chair the debate, with the issues being formally voted on, or will there be more free-ranging discussion to arrive at mutually agreed solutions? In my experience the discursive approach works far better, and on the few occasions when our committee had to resort to formal voting it was a sign that things were not going well. Surprisingly, even when there was discord, voting could not always be relied on to produce the most sensible conclusion. For example, at one of our first meetings there was great disagreement about bar opening nights. To try to resolve this we finally voted on the various alternatives. The result, however, was an unhappy and nonsensical compromise (the bar to be open every night except Thursday) which pleased nobody. It took a few tactful late night phone calls to retrieve us from the mess we had created.

Bear in mind too that most "committee" people enjoy a good argument. The meetings provide a chance for them to show off their eloquence or display how doggedly determined they can be if they choose. For some the fierce discussion in an argumentative committee meeting is like a tough game of squash—it allows them to let off steam at the end of a hard week. So you may find yourself wondering, as a meeting drags on, whether there is a real disagreement over the issues or whether people are simply enjoying the repartee. A skilful chairperson, though not wishing to deprive members of their fun, will curtail unnecessarily protracted banter, so that there is sufficient time for all the items. The discussion of a controversial subject needs strategic placing on the agenda. If it is kept towards the end, when people are itching to get off home, then unnecessary discussion will be kept to a minimum. Alternatively, it has been suggested to me that at the start of a meeting, if antagonistic members are late, the contentious issue should be quickly rushed through, but I do not think I could recommend such devious manoeuvres.

It sometimes happens that despite your best efforts the committee does reach an impasse; the discussion goes round in circles and no agreement can be reached. If you think that voting would not help for the reasons set out above, it may be worth simply postponing the decision so that people have a chance to cool down. To my amazement I sometimes found that within a couple of days after the most heated debate the participants would have forgotten exactly what it was they had been so vehemently fighting for; it would not then be hard to get agreement.

Delegation and motivation

The ability to delegate is one of the most crucial skills for any management role. Unfortunately, it can also be one of the most difficult. Done well and the job becomes a pleasure, but done poorly

and you simply create extra work for yourself. One often hears it said
that if you want something to be done properly, it is no good asking
others, you have to do it yourself. This, I believe, is due to a lack of
understanding about what makes good delegation. It is not fair
simply to expect others to do the boring aspects of a task, which you
cannot be bothered to do yourself; with little interest in it, they will
not care how well it is done or whether it is completed on time. Good
delegation means that people are encouraged to take upon themselves things that they will be good at and will enjoy. It is important
that you entrust them with the task in hand. How they go about it is
up to them, and, though you might have a chat before they begin,
interference from you should be minimal. This is what can make
delegation so hard. It inevitably means your handing over control of
the project, and even if things are not being done how you would
have liked or up to your meticulous standards, you must resist the
destructive temptation to interfere, otherwise you may well end up
being told to do it yourself.

One role of the president that is not often realised is that of
"motivator". To get the best out of your team you must ensure that
they feel appreciated and, very importantly, that they are actually
enjoying being on the committee. It is surprising how effective
home-made chocolate cake can be in encouraging people to attend
meetings on time. And even for the tasks that have been given over
to others, an encouraging phone call will never go amiss. Similarly,
the odd box of chocolates or bunch of flowers to say thanks for doing
a good job is money well spent.

Tactical manoeuvres

With the committee up and running, what other advice is there to
ensure a smooth year in office for the first timer? On many occasions
simple, seemingly small, requests will be made of you: Can we
borrow the disco equipment? Can the rugby club buy a new set of
shirts? Can we have £300 for new computer software? Some people
have a knack of catching you at inopportune moments, but the
temptation to give an answer there and then should be avoided,
especially if the answer would be no. Most people do not like being
turned down, and in such circumstances "the diplomatic delay" is
called for. You proclaim that the suggestion, however bizarre or
outrageous, seems to be eminently reasonable but will have to be
thought about and discussed by the committee. This takes the heat

off. Then two weeks later, the committee having given it full consideration, the request is regretfully turned down. For some reason people find this procedure more acceptable than a straightforward "no" first time round.

"Administrative ping-pong" is another manoeuvre to take the pressure off. It is brought into play when you are being pressed for something, such as a report, which you intend dealing with eventually but not with the speed requested. To stall for time you request further information or another document or a different report, anything in fact, to put the ball back in the other party's court so that they think that the delay is now down to them rather than you. Those who have ever tried to claim housing benefit or rent rebate will appreciate that this technique is performed par excellence by the Department of Social Services. You may feel that this is all rather a waste of time; however, for those occasions when it is not politic to inform the others that they will simply have to wait, the illusion that you are getting on with the job may prove rather useful.

Conclusion

During such a year in office life will often be hectic, and at times the workload may seem overwhelming; no doubt your medical work suffers too. However, with a good team the commitment should also be enjoyable, and I would recommend anyone given a similar opportunity to take it up: the education received will be tremendous.

Further reading

Jay A. *Management and Machiavelli*. London: Bantam, 1974.

II EMPLOYMENT

17 Give a reference

John Stallworthy

Not another request for a reference—the second in this mail, and the third so far this week! If you have been irritated by a similar experience, it merely emphasises your need to make an appointment with yourself and take the time necessary to formulate a policy for the future. Having made one, stick to it, unless the need to improve the policy becomes obvious. A request for a reference means that somebody values your opinion, needs your help, and believes you will be willing to give it. Remember that you might not have been in the position to receive such requests if someone had not written a reference to support your successful application many years ago for a much desired post leading to your professional success. He or she was possibly just as busy then as you are now, and probably busier, so be prepared to repay the debt by writing a reference for someone else.

Not everyone is deserving . . .

Look again at the three requests now awaiting reply. The one for S O Slow need not detain you long. You have had no communication from him since he left your department five years ago, not even a note to bring you up to date on his recent exploits, a curriculum vitae, or a letter to say he was giving your name as a referee. His record may have improved, but five years ago it was not outstanding, and all you remember is that you were no happier to see him leave your team than he obviously was to go. These recollections would not increase his chance of success, so a card from your secretary regretting that you had no information with which to support his application and wishing him well would be a kind way of dealing with this request, and might help him to behave more courteously in the future.

The second request is on behalf of U Twerp. You remember him well for a variety of reasons, not least of which is that he was one of the only twins to work in your team. They did not hold posts simultaneously. The elder brother had shown more initiative than his younger companion, even while still in utero, by arriving in this world 35 minutes before him. Thereafter, he slowly but progressively outpaced him. When the elder Twerp applied successfully three years ago for a senior registrar position in a busy provincial teaching hospital, you gave him such a splendid reference that he was actually congratulated at the selection interview on the support he had received from you. A somewhat sarcastic personal letter you received a few months later from the head of his new department contained the following passage, which temporarily distressed you:

> I have just read once again the reference you sent in support of the application made by Mr B Twerp for a senior registrar post in this hospital. You are obviously not interested in ornithology, and cannot distinguish a swan from a goose. What you said about his clinical ability was reasonably accurate, but he is so allergic to work that you must have seen him in a remission period, if in fact you saw him at all! I thought it only fair that as his former referee you should know that his appointment to this hospital has been a disaster.

Fortunately for both you and him, the younger Twerp does not request a reference for that hospital, but, of course, the challenger of your refereeing ability could be on the selection committee nonetheless. Perhaps in the interests of you both, you should decline the request to give a reference for the second Twerp. Now you have had a moment to think about him, perhaps you would agree that he could not be recommended without some reservation. Following the example of some of the consultants and registrars with whom he has been associated, he has become a rather militant member of the "work to rule" brigade. If your reference mentions this he is unlikely to be appointed, and if it fails to do so you may receive another derogatory letter when the truth is apparent soon after his appointment to a new position. Yes, on second thoughts it would be better not to send a reference for Mr Twerp.

114

. . . but some are outstanding

The third and last request is from Miss A Winner, who is just completing her appointment as registrar in your hospital, and wishes your support for her application to secure a senior registrar post in a much larger department, before going overseas to spend her professional life working in the Punjab in a Christian medical college with heavy clinical and teaching responsibilities. Your only hesitation in writing this reference will centre on the mingled feelings with which it will be written. You are anxious to help a most worthy younger colleague, while at the same time you are sad at the thought of losing her from your department. Your expression of these sentiments will provide more help to the selection committee than would an unnecessary paraphrase of the candidate's curriculum vitae, to which they are more accustomed. They already know the appointments she has held but not the use she has made of them. Your comments on this can be vital. Her dedication and motivation, capacity for work, compassion and genuine interest in her patients, her technical skills, the lucidity and quality of her concise, carefully dated and signed records in beautiful, legible handwriting, and the respect and affection in which she is held by students and professional and ancillary staff are the hallmarks of the excellent doctor you will be unhappy to lose and they should be looking for. Say so in your reference, and remember to comment on her good health record. If she is not shortlisted for interview, the district health authority should review the membership of the selection committee and look for some modern Oslers to replace them.

After these reflections your policy for handling requests for references should be taking shape. To write one should be a pleasure and not an ordeal if you are selective, honest, accurate, relevant, and concise. The result should encourage the selection committee to shortlist the candidate for interview. If this happens, you both will be on trial, with the candidate's performance and your credibility at stake.

18 Write a job description

Ron Firth

A job description is probably one of the most neglected and under-rated documents in employment. When they do exist, job descriptions are often poorly written and out of date. In many instances they are non-existent—strange treatment for such an important document, which, if used properly, should represent the essential foundations on which employer and employee relations are built.

Importance of the job description

Recruitment and selection of staff

At the outset of the recruitment and selection process it is important to have an accurate and up-to-date job description. This gives the recruiter, who is often not directly concerned or familiar with the particular post, an appreciation of the duties and responsibilities of the job and helps in deciding on the most appropriate method of recruitment, advertising media, and interview techniques and, finally, in considering the suitability of the applicants. A job description is also useful for the applicants, giving them a better appreciation of the extent of the job.

Job grading

Any system of job grading, whether formal or informal, relies heavily on the existence of job descriptions, which often provide the most effective means of understanding the extent of duties and the relative values of various jobs within an organisation.

Performance appraisal

In its simplest form an appraisal of performance aims at assessing performance against the agreed duties of the job. Absence of a detailed job description can lead to misunderstandings and uncertainties, which often contribute to poor performance.

Training

In the development of a structured training programme the job description provides a useful starting point in establishing the skills and knowledge required to complete the tasks of the job satisfactorily, and this in turn should help to highlight individual training needs.

Supervisor–staff relations

Often a breakdown in relations can be traced to a lack of understanding of or disagreement about the extent of the duties and responsibilities of a post—a problem that is usually overcome or avoided by the existence of a detailed job description.

Content and format

There is no set approach for writing a job description that is suitable for all jobs. Generally, a more senior and complex job requires a more detailed job description than a junior and fairly simple job. As a general rule, aim at keeping it as brief as possible. Usually only the main duties and responsibilities need to be included.

Although the format varies considerably, most job descriptions cover certain main areas:

(1) Personal and organisational information is given, including the job title, the location of the job and the department, the title of the person to whom the employee reports, and the name of the person who prepared the job description and the date of its completion. If appropriate, the number of people reporting to the employee should be mentioned. In many organisations the name of the current job holder would also be included.

(2) A brief statement—usually restricted to one or two sentences at most—encapsulates the main purpose of the job.

(3) For senior management posts the description usually includes some of the main dimensions associated with the job—for example,

---

ABC Corporation

Job description

Job title Secretary

Department Finance

Relationships
- Immediate supervisor: head of department
- Subordinates directly supervised: none
- Other persons with whom you have regular working contact: all members of Finance Department. Limited contact with members of other departments. Telephone contact with suppliers

Main purpose of the job
- To provide secretarial support to the head of department

Main duties and responsibilities
- Typing of correspondence, memos, and reports
- Keeping diary, arranging meetings, and organising travel
- Maintaining filing and bring forward systems

Education and training and experience required

- GCSE level English and Maths minimum
- Secretarial training and secretarial experience at a senior level
- Confident shorthand—90 words per minute or more (used recently). Word processing skills preferred

---

the number of people employed, the size of revenue, the turnover, and the capital controlled.

(4) The main section of the description identifies the main duties of the job, usually as a detailed list of duties or in narrative form; in both cases the aim is to specify clearly the main tasks.

(5) Many descriptions include details of the qualifications and level of education, experience, and skills appropriate to the job. Although this is more of a "person specification" than a description of the job, it nevertheless fits quite comfortably within a job description, as it helps in forming an overall impression of the job. There is an increasing tendency to include details of certain terms and conditions of employment, such as hours of work, rates of pay, and on-call arrangements, but unless the case for doing otherwise is particularly strong, this type of information should more properly be left to the contract of employment.

(6) In large complex organisations it is often advisable to attach a copy of the departmental or divisional organisation chart as an aid to clarifying precisely where the job fits into the organisation.

Who writes the job description?

There are several options as to who should write a job description, and the determining factor is usually the size and structure of the organisation. A job description may be written by the current employee, by his or her manager or jointly, by a specialist job analyst, or, in some cases, by a committee.

The employee should have a better understanding of the job than anybody else and should therefore be well placed to write the job description. There are, however, several possible pitfalls; the employee may, for instance, be too subjective or may not be doing the job correctly, when the resultant description is probably inaccurate. Although the manager should have the advantage of having an overall view of the job, this may not be sufficiently detailed to do justice to a detailed job description. The joint approach is probably the most effective, the employee preparing a first draft, which is vetted and eventually approved by the manager through a process of open discussion. Of course, in the case of a new job this option would not be available. Larger organisations often employ specialist job analysts, some of whose duties are to write job descriptions. This approach has some obvious advantages, such as consistency, impartiality, and experience, but substantial input by the employee and his or her manager and the authority of the manager for final approval are still advisable. Although rather uncommon, in some organisations job descriptions are written and approved by a committee. This can be cumbersome and should be avoided when possible.

Whatever the system, maximum uniformity of format, terminology, and the amount of detail is important, particularly when job descriptions are used to evaluate jobs or for grading, when there is a danger that the length of the job description will influence its rating. One final point to bear in mind: the job description is intended to describe the job, not the person doing it.

When to write the job description

Ideally, a job description should be completed before the job is filled, but this may not always be possible in a business that is introducing a system of providing job descriptions. In this case the right time is "as soon as is practicable", having first cleared the

---

XYZ Institute

Job description

Job title Librarian   *Location* London

Department Central library

Principal purpose of job
To lead the development of information services in the institute's library

Staff supervised
• Library services manager, three assistant librarians

Responsibility for equipment
• Extensive microcomputing equipment, including DEC Micro Vax 2000, IBM and BBC microcomputers, CD-ROM mass storage device, optical character reader, photocopiers, and other office equipment

Financial responsibilities
• Yearly budget in excess of £250 000
• Capital equipment and library stock (nominal) £800 000

Main duties
• Planning and implementation of policies to provide cost effective library services
• Liaison with librarians of other national and international university and professional libraries to develop strategies of library services
• Initiation and management of new information storage and retrieval projects
• Planning and implementing library routines to achieve optimum utilisation of stock for the benefit of members
• Representing the institute at national and international meetings on librarianship and information science
• Statutory duty (under copyright legislation) to recover costs of providing photocopies; setting up a computer invoicing system to ensure recovery of money owed
• Responsibility for the storage, use, preservation, and refurbishment of old and valuable library books

Education, training, and experience
• Degree or postgraduate diploma in librarianship or information science
• Fellow or associate of the Library Association or equivalent qualification
• Proved ability to initiate and manage information science projects

Prepared by ....   Date ....

---

necessary staff communications and agreed the system and method to be adopted. One word of caution: starting and maintaining an effective system of job descriptions is not easy and requires much effort and a disciplined approach. The potential payoff, however—in terms of greater efficiency, better quality of recruitment and selection, greater job satisfaction, and improved staff relations —makes the investment well worth while.

120

Summary

- Decide on the system best suited to your business.
- Ensure appropriate communication with staff concerned.
- Aim at consistency.
- Ensure maximum involvement of current job holder.
- Keep descriptions as brief as possible.
- Ensure effective maintenance and updating of relevant records.

19 Conduct a selection interview

George Dick

It is unfortunate that the medical profession, apart from those branches involved in the Services, has not devoted more time and research to methods of assessing the characteristics of medical personnel, which might have provided a background for career guidance and appointments and could save hours of time of interview panels; industry is a long way ahead in this field.[1] Be that as it may, the interview panel will remain the main selection device for many years to come.

Interviewing panels

In attending interviewing panels I often used to recall a reproduction in one of my schoolbooks of one of Yeame's paintings, "And when did you last see your father"? This picture shows a party of Roundheads interviewing the little son of a Royalist, while his family wait in fear in case the boy's answers to questions lead to disaster.

While an interview, properly carried out, should be a two-way exchange it must always be remembered that everything is heavily weighted against the candidate.

The numbers on the panel, including a committee officer, should not be more than six or seven, and must include members of both sexes and the candidates' future immediate "boss". Sensible candidates will have met this individual before the interview and will have visited the place of work. They will also have discussed the post with other members of staff, including personnel officers or administrators, one or other of whom may be on the panel (indeed they may have made an order of preference before the formal panel interview).

Preliminaries

As an interview is a two-way process the candidate and the interviewers must be properly prepared. The former has probably been coached for the part, but the latter may require some training[2] in gathering information and in assessing the suitability of candidates for the particular job. Before the interview a careful study should be made of the job description, the curriculum vitae, and the application forms; this will weed out some of the applicants and confirm that the candidates are suitable for interview, for it will be possible to make inferences of their ability, for example, from their attainments, and of their stability and health from observing their periods of unemployment.

If the usual procedure is not known, arrangements should be made with administrative officers to ensure that the candidates arrive at intervals of about 30 minutes and not all at once, and that waiting time is occupied by paying the travelling expenses of the candidates, checking addresses, and providing any additional information, such as the names of the members of the interviewing panel.

Before the candidates are interviewed the chairperson should ensure that all members of the panel have been introduced to each other. The panel must agree on the key qualities and attributes required for the post and on the procedures to be adopted. Each member of the panel should concentrate his or her questions on one particular facet of the job or of the candidate. The chairperson should indicate for how long each candidate should be interviewed and at what time the business should be finished. It is fairest to withhold discussions about the suitability of any candidate until all have been interviewed.

Process

Members of the panel should sit round a table and each should be identifiable to the candidate by a nameplate in large letters which also indicates who they represent (nothing elaborate is required, just a folded piece of stiff paper and written on with a felt-tip pen). Unless all members are well known to the chairperson, a seating list of the panel should be given to or made by the chairperson.

How to start

If it is not practicable for the chairperson of the panel to welcome the candidate with a handshake, he or she should at least stand up when candidates are brought in and invite them to be seated. If I am chairing the panel, I then usually say to the candidate "You probably know a number of the members of this committee, but just let me introduce them to you" and proceed to do so. With a committee interviewing many applicants, it is then advisable to identify each candidate: "You are Dr X and you are applying for the post of registrar in psychiatry at Y Hospital". (This may prevent upset, embarrassment, and a waste of time when the panel discover that they are interviewing the wrong person for the wrong job!)

Next you must let candidates play themselves in; they should be asked some general questions of an open type such as: "*How* did you travel?" "*When* did you leave home?" "*Where* exactly is your hospital?" so that they can hear the sound of their own voice. The chairperson should then explain how the interview will be conducted and should ask if the candidate wishes to add anything to the information that has been provided on the application form—for example, a candidate may have completed an examination for a college diploma since applying for the post. All this leads to candidates developing the confidence to play their part in the act. They should be asked if they have read the job description and have any comments on it, and if it seems to suit their requirements. The chairperson should then invite each member of the panel to interview the candidate.

Questions

It is important that each member of the panel establishes a rapport with the candidate. This will be determined by the type of questions that are asked. An interview can be a very trying experience and nothing is gained by starting it with a question such as "What is the biggest mistake you've ever made, Dr A?" (a favourite stock opening question by a particular surgeon). Stress questions (questions designed to uncover sexist attitudes, for example) can come later if they seem to be indicated; it needs to be clear why they are being asked. To begin with the members of the panel must attempt to get the best out of all candidates and not just from a favourite.

The questions asked to begin with should be open questions, which usually begin with the "Six honest serving men...Their names are *What* and *Why* and *When* and *How* and *Where* and *Who*". They should be aimed at finding out attitudes, experience, and suitability, and should not take the form of a tutorial or a viva for a higher degree, which the candidate may have just recently passed: this, of course, does not mean that clinical questions or recent work should not be discussed in moderation.

Direct questions have their place in establishing or verifying faults on the application form, but it is always more pleasant to try to phrase these questions in an indirect way, not "You returned to Ruritania for one year in 1980?" but, "What did you do when you visited Ruritania in 1980?" "How long were you in Ruritania?" If the members of the panel fail to fill in lacunae, it is important that the chairperson should pick up inconsistencies at the end of the discussions. However, except to protect the candidate, the chairperson and other members of the panel should not talk too much and should refrain from interrupting the candidate's discussion with other members of the panel: their turns will come.

I have already indicated that stress questions play little part in a selection interview unless clearly to identify glaring deficiencies that have been concealed by the applicant. Personal questions on religion, politics, and privilege should be excluded and only those family questions that may relate to housing, schooling, and so on should be considered, and asked of both male and female candidates. However, with proper preparation candidates should have obtained domestic information from the personnel department of the hospital or institute before the interview. "What if", or fantasy questions, can often provide useful data on attitudes. We all have favourite questions of this type. I like to ask candidates where they see themselves in 5 or 10 years' time and also what research they would do if they suddenly received a large grant and technician help: "What is the one thing you would like to discover?"

Evaluating

In deciding the suitability of a particular candidate I have always tried to have numerical scales. The items that I used to score varied according to the post, but could include personality (empathy), qualifications, service experience, research work, specialist and administrative ability; these headings may be subdivided as necessary and each scored 0–4 or 5. In the case of general practitioners the items to be scored should also include premises, organisation, attachments, and partners' share of work load. If this method is proposed, it must be discussed and agreed by the panel before the interviews.

It is always worth making a note of each applicant's appearance even if it is just to help to remember them when attempting to decide the most suitable candidate at the end of a long series of interviews.

Experienced interviewers appreciate how easy it is to make erroneous judgments on appearances: while a patient might fail to relate to a surgeon with blue jeans, it could be ideal dress for a doctor in establishing confidence with a patient with a psychiatric illness.

In the past few years a considerable amount of work has been done by industrial and occupational psychologists and by others on interviewing techniques. Perhaps some doctors (although it should be basic to their training) have missed out (as I had) on much information that is available on this subject. Not only does the interviewer need a framework that can be based on something like Professor Rodger's seven-point plan—attainments, general intelligence, special aptitudes, interests, disposition, and circumstances[3]—but we should be trying to make decisions based not just on impressions. I do not agree with Professor Eysenck's views on the validity of the interview as a selection device: "You may as well toss a coin".[4]

After all the interviewers have asked their questions, candidates should be asked if there are any questions that they would like to ask the chairperson or other members of the panel. Following any further discussions, applicants may be asked if they would accept the post if it were offered to them and either asked to wait to be told the decision of the panel or told that they will receive it by letter in a couple of days. The interview procedure is repeated with all the candidates, but often changing the order in which the members of the panel ask their questions.

Decision making

After all the candidates have been seen, I prefer that their suitability should be discussed by the panel before looking at their references. The chairperson should ask the members of the panel if they consider that any of the candidates should be eliminated without further discussion, and then invite a senior and experienced member of the panel to sum up the qualities of the remaining eligible candidates. After that the other members of the panel are invited to

126

contribute their opinions (the individual with the highest score may not be the winner because of heavily weighted contraindications).

The chairperson should ask for the references to be read and read between the lines (I was told that all references given by Einstein were the same and said "A B is in the running for a Nobel Prize"). Panel members should also try to give the references a numerical weighting. Some referees may have a biased opinion. It is better not to give a reference at all about a particular candidate than to give a damaging one. Such references can follow people around; it should be a rule that photostat copies of references are not made. (Following the "leaking" of what I thought was an honest reference that I gave many years ago, I now try to *read* the references to individuals who have asked me to write one for them.)

After the references have been read, the chairperson should invite one of the senior members of the panel to place the candidates in order of merit. This is discussed in turn by each member of the panel and, if agreed, the job is nearly finished. If there is no clear agreement, there will have to be further discussion. It is best to try to obtain unanimous agreement and it is better to make no appointment than to choose someone who does not really fulfil the requirements of the job.

If the candidates have been asked to wait, the candidate recommended for appointment is often invited back to the committee room after all the applicants have been seen: he or she is congratulated by the chairperson and a starting date may be briefly discussed, but all such details should be left to the officers of the committee to arrange outside the committee room.

I prefer that the candidates do not wait to be told the decision. If the candidate who is offered the job refuses, how does the second choice feel about taking a post at which he or she is considered second best? I think a letter should be sent immediately to the selected candidate and after he or she has accepted the job (by return of post or by telephone) the unsuccessful candidates should then be informed.

Minutes and manners

A minute of the meeting should be kept with the names of the members of the panel and with a short report on each of the candidates based on the framework of the interview. Only by starting to keep such data will we ever progress towards the validation of the panel selection technique. Furthermore, if efforts are made towards a numerical expression of the job profile, comparison can be made with the aptitude and suitability of the applicants,[5] for most validation studies have shown that mistakes in selection are made more regularly than people like to admit. A panel interview, like an examination, is an act; "a two-person drama"; the candidate is trying to put up the best possible appearance and so should each member of the panel. Candidates may be coached for meeting panels of examiners—most of us know quite a number of tricks; some interviewers also require to be coached.

Epilogue

And what about the follow-up? Sometimes one of the candidates with the highest "score" fails to get the job because he or she is too specialised or because of lack of experience in some special requirement or for some other correctable contraindication. In these and in other special cases the regional postgraduate dean or one of the consultant members of the panel should informally let the unsuccessful candidate know that, although first choice of the committee, he or she was not appointed for some particular reason. Help to remedy the defect and encouragement to apply for a similar post should be given: counselling is no part of an interview panel's remit but it is an important epilogue.

1 Occupational Personality Questionnaires, published by Saville and Holdsworth Ltd (3 AC Court, High Street, Thames Ditton, Surrey KT7 0SR); see Selective Tests Purpose-made Personality Questionnaire. *Personnel Management*, 1984; Feb: 47.
2 Bayne R, Fletcher C. Selecting the selectors. *Personnel Management*, 1983; June: 42–4.
3 Highaim M. *The ABC of interviewing*, London: Institute of Personnel Management, 1979.
4 Palmer R. A sharper focus for the panel interview. *Personnel Management*, 1983; May: 34–7.
5 Bolton M. Interviewing for selection decisions. Personnel Library, NFER—Nelson Pub. 10 Daxville House, Windsor, Berks, 1983.

20 Appoint a colleague

M C Petch

Appointing a colleague is rather like choosing a spouse, except that divorce is not really an option. In both cases you may have to live with the consequences of your decision for several decades and you may mistakenly believe that you are in control, whereas in reality there is usually some mother-in-law-like figure manipulating events. Do not be alarmed by this. Arranged marriages can be most successful because neither party has undue expectations of the other. Provided you can live with the other party, the marriage can be made to work and your differences will lead to a stronger unit. My experience of seeing the NHS consultant appointments system in action may help show others how to, or not to, choose a colleague.

These comments apply only to senior NHS appointments, and are being written at a time when the traditional concept of the hospital consultant is being revised. Since the implementation of the NHS reforms district and regional health authorities have disappeared. All hospitals have become self-governing trusts and most are seeking to alter the terms and conditions of service of their employees, including senior medical staff.

The chief executives of trust hospitals have an obligation to provide a quick, economical service in competition with other trusts. The treatments they offer have to have proven medical value. This naturally poses the question "Does the trust really need a highly trained and expensive consultant to provide a routine service for many established cost-effective procedures, for example cataract extraction, hip replacements, prostatectomy, and simple anaesthesia?" Would it not be better for most trusts to employ Calman or

European type specialists with six years' training and have fewer old-fashioned consultants, whose additional responsibilities, such as developing the service, teaching and research, are of little benefit to most trusts? An even more fundamental question is round the corner: "Can some medical procedures be undertaken by people without a medical degree?" Surgical assistants are already here!

The profession faces many challenges but for the moment the NHS Management Executive Report of the Joint Working Party on the Review of Consultants (October 1993) has recommended that senior NHS appointments will continue to be centrally determined and controlled by statute. Trusts can, however, set their own terms and conditions, including short-term contracts. It does seem likely that the traditional consultant, who has, overall, served the NHS very well for the past four decades, will survive.

Preliminaries

The preliminaries take a long time, often a year or more in the case of a vacancy due to retirement. As soon as a close colleague whispers his or her intention of going, start planning. Decide what you want to do because at this stage a short friendly discussion will enable you to take over the desirable parts of your colleague's practice and shed, or at least share, the undesirable parts of yours. Then write down carefully the fixed sessional commitments that must be covered. For a cardiologist this might include two or more clinics, two investigative sessions, three ward rounds, one or two sessions in coronary care, two for management, one for reading and research, one for teaching, one for travel; already the week is overbooked. It might seem obvious to you that there is a pressing need for a replacement but do not be surprised when this is challenged. Write down why a replacement is essential and discuss this and your provisional job description with your department. Be prepared. When your retiring colleague begins to talk about dates, the news will already be widespread and urgent claims for new consultants in other disciplines will be presented from the most surprising quarters.

The details of the job description have to be discussed by the medical advisory committee of your trust hospital, often a consultant staff council. Make sure your friends are there; you may find that you don't have many on the day. If the chairperson at least understands your case, you may get your job description accepted with minor modifications. If the chairperson does not, then the matter will be deferred for a month, and then another month, and so on. If two hospitals are concerned, your task is at least doubled. Eventually a job description must be agreed even though your secretary can spot the flaws. Keep a careful record of these discussions. Many months may yet elapse before the appointment, and during these months people will forget that they ever took place. They may assert later that they did not have the opportunity for comment. To avoid this it is important to ensure that all potentially interested parties see a copy of the job description.

You must involve trust management at an early stage but exactly who you approach, and when, is problematical. Your old-fashioned, helpful, and independent district medical officer is no longer there to give dispassionate advice. The nice, well-informed, mature person in personnel has been replaced by a youthful, "human resources manager" who has a psychology degree. Your chief executive might have done a deal with the next trust to "rationalise" your department. The chairperson of your trust board may not understand. Your local BMA representative may not be very helpful. You should ring round your colleagues in other trusts. They face similar problems, or worse. Not all is gloom, however. In any fixed market where there are losers, there must be some winners apart from the managers. A lot of cardiologists are getting appointed!

At this stage you will also become aware that the senior registrar grapevine is waiting for the advertisement. At meetings colleagues you hardly know will explain that their own time-expired senior registrar is very good and thoroughly worthy of "your" job. Listen politely and question discreetly. Treasure the comments, because as the time of the appointment draws near colleagues will become more elaborate with the truth. Information volunteered casually at a conference dinner is likely to be more accurate than that elicited by direct questioning once the shortlist has been made.

The advertisement

A short conventional advertisement in the *BMJ* and *Lancet* is sufficient. Trust hospitals that take several column inches merely announce their fear that there may be few applicants. If the job is unattractive, then you should have recognised this and taken steps to improve it beforehand. In cardiology, for example, there is a lack of suitably trained senior registrars for consultant posts in district hospitals. A simple and mutually beneficial arrangement may be to

131

link such posts with a specialist centre giving opportunities for cardiac catheterisation, for instance. There are other similar devices to improve a job.

The timing of the advertisement should allow for the following: one month or so before the closing date, a further month for shortlisting (before and during these months an appointments committee will be chosen and a date for the appointment agreed, although this may take longer if one potential member is important and busy), two weeks for the appointment to be confirmed, and then three months for the successful candidate to work out his or her notice. Six months therefore elapse between the appearance of the advertisement and the provision of a service. An interregnum is unsatisfactory but has unsuspected advantages—desks are cleared, clinics dwindle, a locum may shed light on your former colleague's habits, and, of course, the trust may save money.

Trawling for applicants is generally a mistake. A potential applicant who is working overseas may merit a letter and a copy of the job description, but more active canvassing may secure an applicant who is successful and later decides not to take up the appointment or does so only to leave shortly afterwards.

Appointments committee

Consultant appointment committees are still governed by a statutory instrument. Until April 1991 the committee included representatives from the district and regional health authorities, but now the working party has recommended that the committee should be simplified as follows:

- lay person (usually chairperson)
- chief executive of trust
- medical director of trust
- local consultant
- royal college assessor
- other.

The basic number is therefore five. "Other" may include a university representative in the case of a trust with a substantial teaching commitment. Academic appointments themselves should be subject to more liberal guidelines. If two trust hospitals are concerned, then extra members are allowed. If an unrepresented department feels particularly aggrieved, it may be represented by an observer. This new constitution seems fairer and it is to be hoped that the working party's recommendations will be ratified in the very near future.

The choice of members of a traditional appointments committee was largely mysterious and probably undemocratic. But now there is less room for manoeuvre. Nevertheless, the choice of the local consultant, royal college assessor and other, remains vitally important because the flavour of the committee determines the nature of the appointment. The royal colleges and faculties would do well to publicise their selection process. Does the registrar of the Royal College of Physicians, for example, seek and heed the advice of the college's specialist committees?

The members of an appointments committee are responsible for drawing up the shortlist. Most members will make up their list from the submitted applications with no personal knowledge of the candidates. Those members who are going to have to work very closely with the successful applicant need to do more. To see all applicants is very time consuming and may be impossible. To see some seems unjust. To see none is a luxury that only uninvolved members can afford. There is no easy compromise, but all serious candidates should be seen.

Some candidates are exemplary in their organisation. They arrange a visit to suit your convenience, turn up on time, ask a few relevant questions, see the departments, say thank you, and express a wish to come back if they are shortlisted. Others just make difficulties: they will trip you up in conversation, criticise your department to others, ask if the job description can be altered, and may even lodge a complaint against you—all of which are memorable experiences. Usually there are too many of the first group. Your responsibility is to try to treat them all equally, even though you know that you can work better with some.

An NHS consultant is appointed to provide a service in a particular discipline. Unfortunately, this is the one talent that cannot be assessed at an appointments committee. Undue weight is often given to a candidate's research publications. His or her capacity for continued service has to be gauged from informal consultation before the interview. The chief fault with the present system of appointing consultants is the lack of opportunity for assessing a candidate's clinical ability and the likelihood that he or she will continue to provide a service over two decades in the face of such temptations as private practice. Hence the importance of previous informal consultations.

Any curriculum vitae will naturally look splendid. Publications will be there in plenty. But no one will tell you whether these were acquired by evening and weekend work or by delegating clinical duties to registrars and senior house officers. There is a strong case for allowing candidates to list only a few publications, perhaps three presentations, three original papers, and a review article or a book. References from senior medical staff, which are generally presented at the time of the interview, are likewise paeons of praise. What you really need to do is to have a word with an outpatient sister, ward clerk, or medical secretary—namely, someone who can tell you whether a candidate pulls his or her weight. The vast majority do of course; hence such testimonials are regarded as superfluous. There seems to be no good reason why the performance of senior registrars should be judged solely by their seniors; they may be at their best when their seniors are away. Perhaps in future a shorter curriculum vitae should be balanced by more testimonials, including, perhaps, a nurse's, a manager's, or a junior doctor's.

The length of the shortlist is an easy matter; six is too many. Only those applicants with whom you can work over a decade or more and who have the necessary qualifications should be shortlisted.

Shortlisted candidates will usually pay several visits and will generally be invited to attend a "trial by sherry" on the evening before the interview. This dyspeptic experience gives everyone a chance to meet their potential colleague. Let someone else be the host, get rid of the guests and supervise the subsequent discussion while you make notes and watch your current colleagues empty the bottles.

The interview

Everything truly hinges on the interview. Whatever machinations have taken place beforehand are now exposed. The power blocs become apparent. You can only watch with fascination as experienced committee members have their way. You may wish that you had taken more trouble to influence people before, yet to have done so may have laid you open to the charge of trying to fix the job.

There is in practice little opportunity for detailed questioning. If five candidates are shortlisted and if each member spends only five minutes talking to the candidate and an additional five minutes are allowed for changeover, then the interview will last three hours, and this is before any discussion can take place.

These three hours may be a revelation. The candidate that you thought was ideally qualified for the job may be destroyed by subtle questioning. Another may reveal an inadequate understanding of the job despite your careful explanation and job description. A third may admit to liking clinical work but goes home at 6.00 pm to help put the children to bed instead of pursuing laboratory research. The strengths and weaknesses of the committee system are exposed in this most crucial of all committees. The tension is inevitable because so much is at stake and because you and the other medical members will remember the day when your own future career was being assessed in a similar fashion. Unlike every other medical committee, no one nods off.

The order of interviewing and speaking is generally the same; the college representative speaks first, then those least concerned with the job, and finally the trust representatives, including yourself. Usually, and perhaps surprisingly, the decision is immediate and unanimous. Rarely is no appointment made, the usual reason then being that the job is in some way deficient. The fact that so many appointments turn out to be a success may have more to do with earlier selection than the final consultant interview. Senior registrars are a select group of highly talented, industrious, agreeable, and strongly motivated people.

You do not have to ask questions; you will probably have asked all the important ones beforehand. You may wish to ask one or two to clear up any confusion created by other members. Remarkably, other members may be offensive about your department; if you can rise above the temptation to criticise theirs, then you will be proud of yourself afterwards.

Afterwards

You will not know whether you have made the correct choice until at least two, and probably five, years have elapsed, but two things you will know. Firstly, you will feel that there has to be a better method of appointing a colleague. And secondly, you are no longer viewed as the new, energetic, young consultant. Suddenly polite colleagues are describing you as the doyen of the service, while most think of you as quaintly senile.

21 Choose a house officer

John S Yudkin

As with much else in health care in Britain, market forces have a major effect on the process of choosing a house officer. The professorial house surgeon job, or senior house officer rotation in medicine at a district general hospital with a good membership course, is probably going to be more oversubscribed than a psycho-geriatric post in Rejkyavik. If you are in the seller's market it can be quite an ego trip to find so many bright-eyed young people falling over themselves to work for you, even though this is a bit like taking pleasure at being at a slave market. But how do you decide who is the best candidate for the job?

The selection of candidates for a medical job requires receipt of a curriculum vitae plus an interview, a process which has changed little in living memory. Why the medical profession should have been left standing at the lights while industry has zoomed off over the horizon may reflect the innate conservatism of our profession. On the other hand, it seems that the method works reasonably well, and in general the two parties seem to end up viewing the process as reasonably fair (except for those who don't get appointed). This interpretation probably reflects a general unwillingness to dip toes into new and uncharted waters. But you will need to ensure that your selection process is fair, and, increasingly, seen to be so.

What are you looking for?

Different consultants have diverse views about what qualities they want in a house officer. Some are determined to select someone in their own image, a process of cloning that antedated by some years the discovery of reverse transcriptase, and which is helped by the fact that the newly qualified doctor has often acquired many of the attitudes and prejudices of his or her teachers, albeit with a more limited transfer of knowledge and skills. Despite my critical tone, I think the habit may be widespread: my juniors have heard themselves described as radical extremists during the campaign about junior doctors' hours of duty.

The requirements that would be fairly universally accepted, besides a level of knowledge and skill that would make the person competent to perform the routine tasks of everyday practice, are the following abilities:

- to act in emergency situations in an organised manner;
- to know when to ask for help;
- to relate sympathetically to patients, even when pushed or tired;
- to work well with other members of the firm, other health workers, and students;
- to organise the workload, both to facilitate patient care and to permit adequate time for relaxation;
- to learn from observation, advice, and experience, and adapt accordingly;
- to contribute to informed debate, without uncritical acceptance of all dogma.

In essence what you are probably looking for is someone in whom you would happily place your patients' care when you aren't there.

Many of these characteristics are impossible to judge in any way other than by working with the person for the duration of a six-month job. It is, of course, possible that you will have worked with the applicant before, perhaps as a medical student or locum attached to your firm, or in a more junior post in the same hospital, and if so, this simplifies the selection process. The two house physicians I have most liked and respected were both on my firm for their first clinical student attachment, and with each of them it was apparent from the first few days that they would be the sort of doctors in whose hands I would happily put myself if I were ill. Nevertheless, there are many hazards in relying on personal preference, rather than on judgment of skills and abilities, in selecting your house officer.

137

The selection process

The process of choosing a house officer is open to bias and prejudice. It is, happily, no longer acceptable or legal to discriminate on the grounds of gender or race, but doubtless there are still examples of such discrimination in action. Your hospital is likely to have an equal opportunities policy and you may well find yourself contravening this if you are not careful to keep personal prejudice out of the selection process. Many health authorities offer training in selection and interviewing processes and in equal opportunities awareness. Guidelines for selecting, shortlisting, and interviewing include producing an agreed job description, writing specifications of the qualities applicants require for the post, and keeping careful notes on the grounds whereby candidates are excluded, as these would be necessary in any claims against the authority that went to industrial tribunal. This is another area of the selection process in which the medical profession has some catching up to do, but it clearly can no longer consider itself either beyond reproach or beyond recrimination.

The curriculum vitae

If you have a much larger number of applicants than there are posts available you will have to whittle the number down to a shortlist. In general, the application form and curriculum vitae are the first pieces of information you will have about your potential house officer. Candidates surely realise that they can make or break themselves by their application, so it is surprising that the quality of these documents is so variable.

You can learn a great deal about people's characters and suitability for a post by reading a covering letter explaining why they feel that this job is right for them, or a curriculum vitae that gives more than the crudest chronological details of education and previous posts. The quality of the document is also important. The poorly photocopied curriculum vitae, with the last three posts added in handwriting with different inks, gives a poorer impression than one produced on the applicant's Amstrad—and it may be valuable to know that one's potential house officer is computer literate. And talking of literacy, I suspect it is not just my own personal fetish to prefer house officers who can spell.

The content of the curriculum vitae may also be useful. I don't feel that a previous PhD, a BSc, or a list of publications is that important in the selection process at house officer level, where the main function of the job is involvement in patient care. The performance of clinical tasks and the acquisition of knowledge and skills do not seem to correlate well with academic qualifications, and I even have my doubts that the scientific content of BSc courses really instils a more scientific or critical approach in the graduates. Nor, it seems, does the huge variety of experiments across the country in innovative approaches to medical education translate into doctors easily identified as, say, "obviously a Southampton graduate" or "a Bart's chap". The range of characteristics of newly qualified doctors is so wide that any small difference attributable to the medical school would be missed as a type II error, and in any event is more likely a result of differences in admission policy rather than in the course itself. Nevertheless, there may be something on the curriculum vitae, like the medical school, or a hockey blue, or an Arsenal supporter, that you decide is grounds enough for offering the job.

The curriculum vitae should be used to get some view of the applicant's character, and not just to decide that the person should be capable of performing the tasks required. The description of the elective period, of holiday jobs or work experience before medical school, of participation in a student psychotherapy scheme, or of leisure activity will give a more rounded impression. It is, however, quite difficult to know how to react to statements like "My most important personal influences have been Nietzsche and Charlie Parker."

The interview

Although the process of selection by interview has its critics, I feel that it is a valuable way of seeing how you will relate to your potential house officer. There are candidates who are struck mute, or who are clearly terrified by the whole occasion, while others are so laid back about it that they may seem to be trying to put the interview panel at their ease. Although on occasions the former is merely the result of panic at the sight of the panel of 12 senior professionals across a table, or the latter a manifestation of β-blockade, it is my view that the impression given at interview is often the factor that, given that any of the shortlisted applicants could probably do the job well, best differentiates the one person with whom you will most enjoy working from the rest.

In many walks of life the standard interview format is being replaced as the sole selection method, and you may decide that, for example, you would like, in addition or instead, to invite all your shortlisted candidates to spend a half day attached to your firm. The structure of junior hospital jobs, however, may make this difficult to arrange. Another possible constraint is that you may not be selecting a house officer as an individual, but as part of a linked house job scheme, or for a postgraduate training scheme for all senior house officer posts in the hospital, which may impose limits on what is feasible. You may want to see applicants yourself before the interview, ostensibly to let them have a look around and find out about the job, but really to provide the opportunity for a one-to-one discussion. For the selection process itself, even if it is for just your job, it is important not to interview on your own. Another consultant or your registrar can be a useful contributor to help balance bias, and the hospital personnel department may wish to be involved. Even if you don't see them before the interview, it is important to encourage candidates to come to the hospital to have a look around, and if someone else shows them the ropes, and not their potential consultant, the risk of bias can be reduced. The candidate who has seen the hospital and who has spoken to the present house officers is clearly interested in the job.

Interviews can be very boring—for both sides of the table. To sit through a series of 15 sets of "Why do you want to come and work here?" is unlikely to give much insight into personality. On the other hand, an equal opportunities policy means that you should cover the same broad area with each candidate. It is certainly not acceptable, for example, to ask only female applicants what are their plans for a family. In selecting topics it is worth picking up interesting items from the curriculum vitae, quite aside from obvious plants like Nietzsche and Charlie Parker. You will be able to get a good idea of how well the applicants can think on their feet by asking rather less obvious questions—such as "What lessons for the organisation of health care in the United Kingdom did you learn from your elective in the Amazon Basin?" You will certainly find interviews more interesting and the responses more varied if you introduce topics such as ethics, or prevention, or health care structure into the interview. For example, you could experiment by asking the candidates how they might cope with a described case in which there is a conflict of interest about confidentiality, or what they think about the concept of GPs' use of deputising services in the light of campaigns about hours of work. If you are confident in your skills in the performing arts you might even attempt a five-minute role play, although the pale, sweaty, un-β-blocked candidate is likely to be turned into a jibbering wreck by this approach.

The references

At pre-registration level you will probably have references from the subdean of the medical school, and perhaps a consultant for whom the applicant did a student assistantship, but these are unlikely to provide much more insight into character than would a bank manager's reference, and merely attest to medical solvency. At the senior house officer level a telephone call from one of the referees may be more informative than words on paper, although this is increasingly viewed as contravening equal opportunities policies. Phrases like "the best houseman I have ever had" or "a high flyer" abound, but you occasionally still see references like the apocryphal, "Dr X has performed his tasks entirely to his own satisfaction." Many referees are keener to tell you what a good, or busy, job they provide. Others may give you good material for between-the-lines detective work—such phrases as "she has matured in approach during the tenure of this post" or "with supervision, his clinical skills are reasonably safe" may give cause for concern.

Allocating people to jobs

If you are interviewing on your own your first choice will usually be your next house officer. If, however, you are part of a linked house officer scheme your preference list may be subjected to a process of computer matching. It is remarkable how much acrimony this seemingly objective process arouses, with paranoia in the district general hospital that some third-to-first choice matches are more equal than other first-to-first matches (especially if the former is on the professorial unit). It is, however, equally likely that dissatisfaction will ensue from the computerless panel interview. In our hospital the senior house officer interviews, which take place every six months, produce a surprising degree of consensus on who should be appointed, but with much cattle trading on who gets allocated to which job. You might discuss with your colleagues approaches such

141

as rotating the option of first choice, for example, to the shortlisters, or, unless you are the most junior, giving the senior consultant first option. It should be possible for the candidates and the consultants all to write down their first three choices and to attempt a point scoring system, but the matching process may take a very long time without a computer.

Conclusion

When I was originally asked by the former editor of the *BMJ* to share my expertise in this area, I felt that it would be far easier to write a *How To Do It* on something where the correct performance of the task could be readily evaluated. I would be happier, for example, writing about how to give insulin—but perhaps choosing a house officer needn't be so different. Except that in the former case you'd use a needle, not a pin.

22 Assess a job

A J Asbury

Sooner or later the doctor has to apply for jobs, and this chapter deals with the problem of assessing a new post. The information is intended as a prompt so that applicants will remember to ask the relevant questions. Obviously some matters will be of greater interest to consultants than to junior staff, and vice versa.

The campaign

Unless times are particularly hard, one should always consider a new post as the next step in a well-organised campaign to get to your career goal and therefore each move should have objectives that you must fulfil. This may be, for example, additional training in a medical specialty, or a lighter job to give you time to read for an examination, or possibly a jumping-off post where you can acquire useful referees to get your consultant post. Time spent discussing your career plan with a local specialty adviser will be well repaid, as will careful study of the current and future workforce market.

Be prepared

The bush telegraph that permeates the medical world usually gives warning that an interesting post is likely to be available, and this is the time to start your preparation. Use the library to find out about the staff, the hospital itself, and the local trust situation. Are there any special facilities, "big names", suitable referees, etc? The *Medical Directory* can give a good clue as to the ages of staff and allow

143

an estimate of when people will retire. If your plan requires certain people to be your future referees then estimate their age to make sure they will still be around when you need them for the next step.

First contacts

You should already be looking out for the advertisement, and as soon as it appears ring up and get the details and an application form. Also request general details of the hospital trust, and ask for a specimen contract. With the advent of trusts, it has become very important to read your contract carefully, and if you don't understand any aspects, get advice early by ringing your local BMA office. Apart from saving yourself the embarrassment of looking foolish at an appointment committee when asked about the contract, you might find that some details of the contract are negotiable, and negotiation always requires preparation.

Make arrangements to visit the department, and emphasise that you would like to talk to several people, and look round. Try to avoid Friday visits, as people may be away at meetings. You will have to make specific appointments to see, for example, the chairman of the directorate, the local service organiser, and the relevant managers. The titles of the crucial people may vary; if in doubt, seek advice from a colleague from your specialty actually working in the hospital. The more senior the post, the more people you must meet.

When the details arrive, compare them with your career plan. If they fit in, then complete the application form and your curriculum vitae in the style requested. Don't forget to ask your referees for their permission before quoting their names and do supply them with copies of your curriculum vitae. Depending on how the closing date for applications fits in with your visit, you may be able to avoid posting your application and be able to deliver it by hand when you visit.

The list

Start your preparation for your visit by assembling a list of questions, remembering that some things are better asked of an administrator and some of medical staff. Use the items below as a prompt, and expand and modify the list according to your own interests and requirements.

Finance: income

What is the salary? How might your salary vary with the work of the trust? When would you get your next increment? Are there other sources of income—for example, cremation fees, visits, etc? Will you get your moving expenses and other financial assistance that doctors normally expect? Are there possibilities for private practice? How is the private practice organised?

Finance: expenses

Will you be able to afford the sort of accommodation that you require? Remember to consider the house prices. What is the likely cost of travel to and from work? Are you expected to pay for parking at the hospital? Will there be school fees and other additional expenses related to children's education?

In the changing climate of the health provision, when checking on one's likely financial situation, ensure that not only are you entitled to a certain benefit, but that it will actually be given.

The job

Does the post give you what you need for your career plan? Does the post carry the required accreditation with the relevant supervisory bodies? Ask particularly about specialty rotations, as these can be very deceptive. For example, you may discover that certain parts of the rotation will be available only when you have completed all the less attractive parts. You may find rotations where access to certain parts is restricted to local trainees. It is important to discover who really controls the rotation, and what sort of say you have in your assignment.

Inquire carefully about the exact nature of the work. Remember "extensive paediatric surgery experience" can mean lots of hernias in children farmed out by the teaching hospital.

Check carefully on the on-call system. Find out how flexible it is; you might need extra flexibility to attend a professional course. What happens in the case of sickness? Do you have to live in when on-call, and if so, is any payment for accommodation required? Is the accommodation reasonable?

Further education in post

Will you be allowed to attend a relevant professional course in the neighbourhood, and will you get your expenses? Will this still hold if

145

there are staffing problems? Will you be allowed to attend the relevant conferences, and will your expenses be paid?

Research

What facilities are there for research? Is research actually encouraged or is it considered to be an annoying necessity? Will you be given time off to do a project relating to your work? Is there somebody to type the manuscript, or can you have access to a word processor? Are there facilities to get bits of equipment made? Is there enough space to store equipment? Is there somebody to give advice on statistical and scientific aspects?

The future of the post

If this move is to be your last before retirement, it is important to consider the implications of current and future government policy for the post—for example, is the trust due to be merged with another? Could the on-call arrangements change so that a consultant is first in line?

The visit

Remember that though this is not "the" interview, it is a time for mutual appraisal, and it is important that you present yourself well. It is definitely the time to dig out the "funeral and wedding suit" and give it a trial run before the interview. In the atmosphere of the informal visit you may well have a better chance to make a good impression than at a formal interview. Don't underestimate the value of the visit; use it well!

Take a spare copy of the job application and your curriculum vitae with you, and if you have written papers, take some reprints; this is often a good "conversation starter". Don't forget your "prompt list".

Take some food with you; many hosts ply you with endless cups of coffee but forget that you have been on a train for four hours before you arrive, and make no allowance for hypoglycaemia.

Make sure that you arrive on time in spite of industrial action on the railways, buses, and so on. Remember that it can take ages to find a department in a big hospital; it may even be in an annexe two bus rides away. Make sure you have time to freshen up before the appointment.

Arrive at the appointed place at least five minutes early, and introduce yourself to the secretary. When you are introduced to your host, make sure that he or she has got your full name correct; you don't want any good impressions to be wasted on another candidate with a similar name. For the same reason try to be sensibly memorable, so that your host remembers you at the interview "Oh yes, he's the one who plays jazz on the trumpet".

When you talk to your host, remember that you are a guest, and try not to conduct an interview, but ensure you cover all points of importance. Few people will object if you say "Do you mind if I make some notes while we talk?" Don't forget to thank your host; he or she may have cancelled a game of golf to see you.

When you have an opportunity to talk to other members of staff, try to establish whether they are happy in their work, since this might indicate your future state. Beware of the person who is very discouraging. This individual might be doing you a favour—or have a sister applying for the same post, or just be one of those people who does not fit in anywhere. Cross-check the meaning of the job description with staff actually in post.

If you are reasonably pleased by what you see and are confident that you want the post, then place your application in the hands of the administration department. At least with the receipt in your hand you can be sure that it has arrived safely. If you are not sure, then send the application later by post, preferably by recorded delivery.

As you leave the area it is worth getting a local newspaper to get an indication of the local house market, and the names of estate agents. Once you have got the names of estate agents from a newspaper, you can always phone for details from home. It is often worth buying a local map, particularly if you are reasonably confident of a move.

As soon as you can, probably in the train, complete your notes on the visit. There may be several weeks between your visit and the interview, and inevitably some details will be forgotten, so keep your thoughts and impressions safe on paper. Even if you do not apply for the post, your notes may be valuable later when a similar post comes up.

Back to the referees

After your visit it might be helpful to discuss the post personally with your referees. They may well appreciate information that would help them to write the most fitting reference.

147

Finally . . .

As medical unemployment grows, competition for posts increases, and the well prepared will have a definite advantage, particularly if they make the best use of the informal visit.

23 Prepare a curriculum vitae

Eoin O'Brien

> *Name, address. Excuse the fantasy.*
> *Photo of the woman I was at twenty.*
> *Marital status: no second finds me the same.*
> *Virgin, mistress, single and married —*
> *Must I conform to a particular brand?*
>
> Patricia McCarthy, *Curriculum Vitae*

I owe a debt of gratitude to a wonderful secretary who once worked in the offices of a Midland dean of postgraduate studies. Having kindly typed my application for a registrar post, she remarked in her characteristically forthright way, "This could belong to any old fool. Let me rewrite it for you". When she presented me with her interpretation of my medical prowess, it took me some time to accept the metamorphosis. I had been given an astute practical lesson. It is, indeed, a sad reflection on our medical schools that we should emerge brimful of matters medical after six years, but untutored in the art of acquiring an appointment—a tedious business that may occupy much of our time. Thanks to my mentor, I am now able to see things from the other side of the fence, and I realise that I was not the only one unable to prepare a curriculum vitae. The standard of CVs submitted for posts at all levels is often abysmally low. At times one is left wondering if the applicant has any schooling in the rudiments of English spelling and writing.

There are many ways of planning a curriculum vitae, and the method proposed here is a personal choice. There are other methods and styles every bit as acceptable. The style chosen, however, should

149

General and personal

Name...

Address ....

Nationality................ Date of birth........... Family ....

Interests ....

General education ....

Undergraduate career

Medical school ....

    Date of entry.................... Date of graduation...

Teaching hospitals..

....

....

Distinctions ....

....

Postgraduate career

Qualifications

Previous appointments

Present appointment(s)

Career plans

Publications (Papers, abstracts, book chapters, papers in press)

Scientific communications (Full presentations, poster presentations)

Learned societies

Referees

Fig 1 Suggested layout for a curriculum vitae

have order and be neatly laid out. It is important to comply fully with the instructions for applicants; if 20 copies of a curriculum vitae are requested, 20 copies must be submitted, however unreasonable this may seem to the applicant. Likewise, if a photograph is requested, one must be supplied. Applications must reach the right person before the closing date. Allow plenty of time for delays in the post and in the hospital distribution of mail.

General presentation

Many hospital authorities make it difficult for the applicant by providing a totally inadequate application form. The best way of dealing with this problem is to submit your own curriculum vitae (fig 1) and to complete the hospital application form only to draw attention to the appropriate page of the curriculum vitae. Sometimes the application form seeks information that would not normally be

150

included in the curriculum vitae—for example, previous salaries. The advice of your consultant or a colleague may be invaluable.

Details

Interests

List your general interests. These might be considered under the headings "cultural", "sporting", or "recreational". Any distinctions in these general pursuits should be briefly mentioned—a cap in rugby, for example, or a place in the college or university debating society.

General education

Schools attended, examinations taken with results, and distinctions should be listed briefly.

Undergraduate education

The date of entry to and graduation from medical school, and all honours and distinctions should be listed. It is surprising how often applicants fail to mention an honours in an examination, or a placing in a prize examination. If there has been a genuine reason for failing or postponing an examination, particularly if this has resulted in a delay in graduation, the circumstances should be briefly indicated— for example, family illness preventing the taking of finals on schedule. If, on the other hand, there are no mitigating circumstances, the dates should merely be stated.

Qualifications

List full titles of degrees and fellowships with dates of award.

Previous appointments

Previous appointments should be in chronological order. It is best to put designation of the post on the left side of the page, the tenure on the right, and a summary of experience beneath this, using the unwritten headings "service commitment", "teaching", "research", and "administration" as appropriate to maintain order and to help you to remember past experience.

Senior house officer to

Professor Oblong,	July 1992–June 1993
Department of Medicine,	(12 months)
University of Maydell and	
St Magdall's Hospital	
London	

Professor Oblong was professor of medicine at the University of Maydell. His special interest was gastroenterology. There were 40 general medical beds and 10 gastroenterological beds. The hospital was on-take one night in four and I was on call one night in three. I gained experience in acute medical emergencies, including acute coronary care. I assisted at Professor Oblong's outpatients twice weekly, at which 2000 general medical problems and 2000 gastroenterological problems were seen annually. I was trained in endoscopic procedures, liver and intestinal biopsy techniques, and was competent to perform these procedures without supervision at the end of my appointment.

St Magdall's is a teaching hospital at which 300 medical students attend. I gave two senior and one junior tutorial to the students each week and participated in the professorial department's clinical teaching sessions, which were held three times weekly, and also at the weekly CPC. I gave six lectures to nurses each term and took part in the general practitioner postgraduate luncheon meetings.

I participated in a trial of a new H_2 antagonist, and assisted at experiments to determine the efficacy of the drug on canine gastric secretion. As a result of this work there has been one publication (see publications), and another is being prepared for submission.

Fig 2 Sample entry for previous experience

Present appointment(s)

The layout is similar to that for previous appointments. There may be, or previously have been, more than one post; for example, if one is or was registrar in medicine and tutor to the medical school, deal with each post separately. In the example shown (fig 2) the greater emphasis is on a service commitment. This would not be the case in an application for a research or tutor's post. For more senior posts administrative experience would become relevant.

Publications

Accuracy in listing your publications is important. Interviewers often check publications—more to familiarise themselves with the standard and content of the work than to verify its existence—and, understandably, a poor view will be taken if the publication cannot be located. Full details of publications should be given in the Vancouver style: each author, the full title, the title of the journal or book, the place of publication and the publisher (books only), the year, volume, and page numbers. An asterisk may be used to indicate those publications in which your contribution was a major one, and this may be indicated in brackets at the head of the list. When publications become more plentiful in the course of time, they should be classified as original papers, abstracts, editorials or leaders, book chapters, reviews, letters (only those that contribute to the literature should be cited), and miscellaneous writings.

Learned societies and committee membership

Mention not only learned medical societies but also cultural bodies that may indicate your involvement in the arts or community affairs. However, if you do list the Forty Foot Bathers Association, be prepared to expound on the qualities that justify its inclusion as a learned society. Committee membership serves as an indication of your administrative experience, and if you have served as chairperson or secretary this should be stated.

Scientific communications

List scientific communications only if you have personally delivered the address. Presumably, if you are a participant in work being presented by another member of the department, your contribution will be acknowledged when the address is published as an abstract or scientific paper. The full title of the address, and the name, date, and venue of the symposium or meeting should be given. Poster displays at major scientific meetings are often published in abstract form and would therefore appear under the list of publications, but it is reasonable to indicate experience in this form of presentation by putting the title of the poster with the place and date of the meeting followed by a note indicating the appropriate publication. (Avoid the temptation to fatten your curriculum vitae by making one piece of work appear at first glance as a number of separate contributions. It is, however, quite reasonable to indicate the progress of a piece of research through different phases of development, for example, from presentation at a local meeting to presentation, perhaps as a poster, at an international scientific meeting, to publication as an abstract, and finally to full publication as a scientific paper.)

Referees

Referees are essential to all applications for jobs and it is important to choose a referee who will speak well of you. Some doctors have a habit of asking for an open reference on completion of a post but this

153

Dear . . .

I wish to submit my application for the post of Senior Registrar at St Margaret's Hospital. I enclose a copy of my curriculum vitae and the names of two referees.

Yours sincerely

Fig 3 Sample covering letter

will usually be refused, and if given is not worth the paper it is written on. Permission to use a referee's name should always be sought in writing *before* submitting the application. Occasionally, time does not permit this and a telephone call may have to suffice, but this should be the exception to the rule. Always give referees details of when you worked for them—they may have forgotten all about you! It is a good policy to let each referee have a copy of your curriculum vitae. Also give details of the post for which you are applying, and the likely date of interview (if the referee is away, the secretary will let you or the interview board know). An interview board is not impressed if the named referees have not sent references, and usually the fault rests with the applicant, who has not allowed sufficient time for the preparation, typing and delivery of the reference. Allow at least three weeks between the time of posting a letter of request to your referees and the interview.

Covering letter

A handwritten letter should accompany all applications (fig 3).

Typing and printing

With the advent of the word processor the task of keeping a curriculum vitae up to date has been made much easier. Once a curriculum vitae is on a disk, it can be updated with ease for each job application without the trouble and expense of retyping the entire document. For doctors well advanced in their careers the task of committing what may be a substantial tome to the disk may appear daunting, but as curricula vitae are demanded not only when a change of appointment is contemplated, but also for grant applications, pharmaceutical trials, and membership application for learned societies, the effort will be well rewarded. Moreover, if one's career is productive, it is surprising how easily publications and achievements are omitted unless they are entered regularly, say on an annual basis.

In the first edition of this book doctors applying for senior posts were advised to have their curricula vitae printed. This expensive exercise is now no longer necessary. With skilful use of the word processor, a tastefully designed and error-free curriculum vitae can be produced inexpensively. A laser or equivalent printer should be used to provide a high-quality typeface. The curriculum vitae can then be photocopied on top quality paper, and for senior appointments the additional small cost of professional photocopying and binding in hard papers is worth while.

Conclusion

Writing a curriculum vitae is a difficult but important task. Do not leave it until the last minute when that friendly secretary you had in mind is the popular choice of your colleagues who are also seeking new jobs. A slovenly curriculum vitae may be judged as the product of a disorderly individual and an indication of performance. If such is not the case, the error for the misconception is entirely one's own; if, on the other hand, the temperament of the applicant is indeed a trifle lacking in discipline and order, the composition of a curriculum vitae may serve as the first exercise in correcting that defect.

24 Be interviewed

James Owen Drife

Taboo for many years, interviews have come out of the closet—at least as a subject for medical articles. Several doctors have offered hints for both candidates and interviewers in articles that are well worth a detour to your local library; thanks to our professional conservatism the advice of past decades remains equally valuable today.[1-9] You may feel that cold-blooded preparation for such a personal affair is unBritish, or that it may even deaden the spontaneity of your performance. However, an interview, like parturition, can be more painful when you don't know what to expect, and you should be better able to relax and do yourself justice if you know the format and some of the pitfalls. Don't be diffident about asking advice from senior colleagues, but be prepared for bland or enigmatic replies, as they may be reluctant to dogmatise in this delicate area. Ignore the anecdotes of your contemporaries: with interviews, as with postoperative complications, those with most experience are not necessarily best qualified to give advice.

I have now moved to the other side of the table, but even now that it is a chore rather than an ordeal, the interview is still taken seriously and is never the mere formality it sometimes seems in retrospect. Some candidates appear well armed with qualifications and experience but do not fit into a committee's plans for a post. A "sitting" candidate may have an appreciable advantage if he or she is well liked, but even the most popular of "home" candidates court disaster if they ignore the rules of the game. Don't be overawed if you find yourself competing with a "home" candidate: if you are on the shortlist, assume the job is there for the taking.

A heterogeneous committee

Appointment committees for hospital jobs vary in size, tending to become larger along the journey from student's bench to regius chair. "Guidelines" exist about their composition for lower-grade posts, and there are statutory regulations at consultant level, but in general the committee will include representatives from each hospital concerned, a member from another district, a lay person, and (for higher appointments) a contingent from the local university and someone from the appropriate royal college or, in Scotland, from the National Panel of Specialists. The meeting is arranged by harassed administrators and the chairperson may not know who the other selectors are until a day or two beforehand. As well as representing different—and even conflicting— interests, the members often vary greatly in seniority. How can the candidate impress such a heterogeneous group of people?

A few generalisations will apply. You should dress to reassure, not to provoke. By most people's standards doctors are quiet and conservative, and interviewees should dress soberly without gratuitous flamboyance such as suede shoes and bow ties. However, within the narrow limits of medical acceptability it is a good idea to stand out a little, and a useful compromise for men is the shameless wearing of a club tie—ideally, a university blue—as a conversation piece. This is recommended only if the candidate is entitled to wear it. If you are a woman you will have worked out, during your years of undergraduate exams, the mixture of femininity and professionalism that suits you best.

When you enter the room you should, in the words of one surgeon, "Go in looking as if you're going to enjoy it". This does not mean entering like a soprano taking an encore at Covent Garden, but it does mean looking a little more relaxed and assertive than you would for a viva exam. Don't worry if you blush or tremble perceptibly: interviewers are familiar with the effects of the autonomic nervous system, and allow for them. You should sit in a businesslike attitude, and your manner should be friendly and alert with just a whiff of authority—similar, perhaps, to the impression you think you give when talking to patients. Look first at the chairperson of the committee, who will try (not always successfully) to put you at ease.

Questions and answers

Answering the questions themselves is simple—in theory. All you have to do is project the right mixture of confidence (without bumptiousness), charm (without sycophancy), intelligence (without being overpowering), good humour (without hilarity), enthusiasm (without recklessness), honesty (tempered at all times with tact), and maturity (without senescence). Answers should be neither brusque nor loquacious. Balance is all important. Generalisations like these trip too easily off the tongue, like speeches at a prizegiving, and it might be more helpful to give examples of specific questions.

Candidates for junior posts will be asked in which direction they see their careers developing and why. Candidates for lecturer posts will be asked if they want to become professors. Women candidates will be asked quite pointedly about the role of women in medicine. Candidates who have switched specialties will be asked about the role of orthopaedics in psychiatry, or whatever the relevant change was. You will be asked what attracted you to the job, and about any unusual features (such as unexplained gaps) in your curriculum vitae. Most committees will ask about research that the candidate has done or intends to do. Candidates for more senior jobs will be asked about recent government reports relevant to their specialty. These are bread-and-butter questions and the way to get them wrong is to look as if you are working them out from basic principles without having thought about them before.

Interviewers are interested in what makes a candidate tick. It is not unknown for interviewees to be asked if they smoke or whether or not they go to church. Surprising importance may be attached to hobbies and interests outside medicine, but be careful to avoid giving the impression that these interfere with your work. The committee wants you to reveal something of your personality, so take the opportunity to talk frankly about your virtues.

There may be trickier questions intended to impress the rest of the committee with the questioner's sharpness as well as test the candidate. In general the interviewers want to help you relax, but if people on the shortlist seem identical in competence and pleasantness it is legitimate to try to grade them according to their response to demanding questions. "What is your weakness?" "What is wrong with your present job?" "If you were given *unlimited* funds for any kind of research, what would your priorities be?" There are no right answers to the heavier questions, but the candidate who makes a tart or glib reply is unlikely to stimulate a spontaneous round of applause. Keep cool by reminding yourself that only the better candidates are asked the most difficult questions, and if you are struggling, remember that other members of the committee will be sympathising as you try to cope with their difficult colleague.

Putting yourself across

In times of difficulty platitudes often reveal their deep meaning, and I have to include advice that may seem hackneyed but bears repeating. Be courteous. Be honest: it is futile to try to put over an insincere impression. Memorise what you have written in your curriculum vitae. Look as if you are interested in that particular job, and not as if you are there simply because you want promotion. It goes without saying that you will have visited the department before the interview—such visits are *not* regarded as "canvassing"—and if you meet a member of the committee at your preliminary visit, the impression you create then may be as important as that at the formal interview. At the end of the interview you will be asked if you have any questions: don't ask about pay or holidays. It is acceptable, and indeed desirable, to have no questions.

The kind of advice given here has been criticised[10] for encouraging "yes men". Committees say they like candidates to state their opinions and defend them, but in fact they do not like such defences to be too successful. I have assumed that you are going to your interview because you want the job, and that it is not a kamikaze attempt to change the interviewers' attitudes to life. Your aim should be to convince the committee that you would be a delightful colleague: if you realise you would find them intolerable to work with, you need not accept the job if they offer it to you. The interview is not, in fact, a battle for survival but a courtship ritual: for the unsuccessful suitors there will be other, often more attractive, opportunities, and for the lucky winner the hard work is just beginning.

1 Rhodes P. Interviews: sell yourself. *BMJ* 1983; **286**: 706–7.
2 Rhodes P. Interviews: what happens. *BMJ* 1983; **286**: 784–5.
3 Oldroyd J. Finding a practice. II: The interview. *BMJ* 1981; **282**: 371–2.
4 Cohen B J. How to interview candidates. *BMJ* 1983; **286**: 1867–8.
5 Sturzaker H G. Survival of the fittest? *BMJ* 1979; **ii**: 374–5.
6 Zorab J S M. Applying for an appointment in anaesthesia. *Anaesthesia* 1980; **35**: 601–6.
7 Giltson A. Applying for an appointment in anaesthesia. *Anaesthesia* 1980; **35**: 1217–18.
8 Proteus. How to apply for medical posts. *Lancet* 1949; **i**: 34–6.
9 Stewart R H M. On the art of being interviewed. *Lancet* 1971; **i**: 127–9.
10 Baumslag N. The pursuit of preferment. *Lancet* 1971; **i**: 596–7.

25 Apply for part time senior registrar training

Jacqueline Morrell, Angela Roberts

Part time training is a valuable career option for men and women, but it is taken up most frequently by women with young children. Two large surveys of doctors showed widespread support for part time posts,[1, 2] even though Warren and Wakefield found almost half their respondents believed part time training to be difficult either to organise or undertake.[2] A report by Isobel Allen, commissioned by the government in 1988, highlighted the second-class image of part time workers.[3] This problem also emerged in work with doctors conducted by Proctor[4] and Gath,[5] although they found the women they studied to be well qualified, motivated, and aiming for consultant posts.

The structure for setting up a part time training has operated in various forms for more than 20 years.[6] However, the first part time general surgical trainee has only recently been appointed. The regulations once known as the mysterious PM(79) have been replaced by "Flexible Training: Senior Registrars", a revised scheme introduced in 1993. This scheme summarises arrangements for the establishment of training posts for doctors and hospital dentists able to work only part time for reasons of domestic commitments, disability or ill health. It requests health authorities to give every encouragement to such doctors and dentists returning to the NHS. Here we will deal only with senior registrar training. A new simplified scheme for part time registrars has also been adopted.

How the scheme works

Part time training opportunities are available in all specialties and there is manpower control to ensure that it is "neither easier nor harder" to obtain a part time post than it is to train full time. There is competition between candidates and the same criteria apply to part time and full time applicants.

The Department of Health advertises the scheme every year and receives quotas from the central manpower committee on the number of posts to be allowed in each specialty. The numbers are collated quarterly; in July 1994 there were 461 part time trainees in England and Wales out of a possible national quota of 634 places. Only four of these were men. Some specialties, such as anaesthetics and psychiatry, were heavily subscribed and had slightly higher uptake than their allocated quota. Many other specialties, including audiological medicine and occupational medicine, had few or no flexible trainees at senior registrar level. There were only 18 flexible trainees throughout all the surgical subspecialities, which had an overall quota of 58 places. This is despite the push made by the Royal College of Surgeons and the Department of Health to promote *Women in Surgical Training* (WIST), and probably reflects in part the deep rooted prejudices of the profession to combining career advancement with domestic commitments.

There appears to be widespread ignorance about the scheme and a lack of preparedness for dealing with candidates that can cause great frustration. Below is a detailed point by point description of the steps an applicant needs to take, followed by some tips gleaned from our and others' experiences. The application procedure involves three steps: manpower approval, educational approval, and funding.

Making an application

Firstly, ensure you are at the right stage to consider higher training: have you the relevant professional qualifications and experience, or are you already in a substantive senior registrar post? Next, decide on a centre for training and draft your curriculum vitae. Make key contacts to obtain support and information:

- dean of postgraduate medicine in the region;
- designated person at the royal college responsible for part time training in your specialty to discuss educational approval (obtain the name of the college specialty adviser while talking to the college);

161

- college specialty adviser in your region to plan an outline for your proposed training programme;
- designated person in the medical staffing division of the regional health authority to discuss the possibility of funding;
- previously successful applicants now training part time in your region for general tips.

Decide on the number of sessions you want to work. The minimum is five and the maximum nine. If you are uncertain it is best to consider starting at a higher level, as sessions may be dropped, but it is hard to increase them. Some "on call" may be required, depending on your chosen specialty.

Manpower approval

Look out for the Department of Health advertisement in the *BMJ* in August or September. Applicants are asked to send their curriculum vitae with a letter setting out reasons for wishing to train part time to the postgraduate dean of the region in which they wish to train. The closing date is 31 October; no applications are considered after that date. If you are already in a full time senior registar post, manpower approval can be made at any time and should be automatic.

The regional postgraduate dean will invite you to interview to consider your eligibility for higher traning and give written endorsement of your application. If the dean does not feel able to support you, then he or she will advise you why, and you should consider reapplying the following year. The dean should also give some idea about the likelihood of obtaining funds.

It rests with the postgraduate dean to ensure you are eligible for higher training. Your curriculum vitae will be sent to the next appointments committee for full time senior registrar posts in your specialty in your region and you will be shortlisted with the full time applicants. You will be invited for interview only if it is felt that you are of equivalent calibre to the others on the shortlist. Should there be no such interview sheduled in the next five-month period (that is, before 31 March), you will be invited to interview in an adjacent region or a special appointments committee will be set up.

At the interview you will be assessed by the same panel that sees the applicants for full time posts and your performance will be considered in relation to them. However, if you are attending for interview out of your own region, arrangements will be made for a consultant from your proposed training scheme to join the appointments committee.

The panel are instructed by Department of Health guidelines to grade you in the following way:

Grade A Outstanding and better than candidates normally appointed to full time posts;
Grade B Of equivalent standard to full time appointees;
Grade C Falling below level required.

Should there be more than one part time applicant, you will be ranked against each other. (It is not clear, however, to what extent the part time applicants should be considered in relation to a "national average" for full time applicants or compared to those full time senior registrars appointed to local training schemes. It could be that potential part time trainees are penalised in their application to prestigious schemes that have high numbers of first class applicants.)

Following interviews, the postgraduate dean will be informed of allocated manpower approvals. He or she then informs the Department of Health of the names, grades and ranks of each part time applicant as soon as possible after 31 March. Manpower approval will not be allocated to those graded C. If there are more suitable applicants than training places available, a waiting list will be established, with preference being given to the highest ranked candidates. Applicants already on a waiting list will take precedence over new applicants. Thus there is no longer the need for trainees to apply every year.

Educational approval

Inform your college regional adviser of manpower approval and arrange a meeting to complete the detailed proposal for your training rotation. This should cover a period of time equivalent to four years' full time work by approximate prorating.

Ensure the clinical tutor submits the detailed proposal to the relevant higher training committee of your royal college for educational approval. These committees meet infrequently, so the timing may be crucial to avoid unnecessary delay. Successful candidates will be able to take up their duties as soon as an agreed training and funding have been arranged.

163

Funding

Meanwhile return to the regional health authority, which will have been informed automatically of your manpower approval by the Department of Health. Contact the regional specialist in community medicine responsible for medical staffing to request funding. Funds do not come from the Department of Health, as is the popular misconception, but from the region itself. The regions differ widely in their willingness to fund part time posts, but each region has a directive from the Department of Health to establish a budget for flexible training.

If funding is not agreed, contact the Department of Health to inform it of your difficulties and to request an extension of manpower approval, as it lasts only for nine months. Then write to, and try to gain support from, anyone who is interested. This could include the postgraduate dean, the college specialty adviser, the reginal chairperson, your royal college, and even the secretary of state for health.

Important points

- Remember it is all down to you. No one else takes responsibility for the overall organisation or coordination of the process.
- Be careful not to miss the deadline for application. The adverisement in the *BMJ* appears only once a year and missing it will mean a long delay.
- In the past, the procedure has not been uniform. Regions have differed in their approach and although recent changes may have improved the system you still need to find out how it works in your region.
- Keep a copy of all correspondence about the application and maintain close contact with your college regional adviser for support and advice.
- Remember, it is a long haul and there is no assurance of funding even if manpower approval is granted. Therefore do not pin your hopes on it or rule out other possible jobs. Look for alternative employment such as job shares, locums, or clinical assistant posts in the meantime in order to survive financially during the procedure.
- Although experience in clinical assistant posts will not be recognised by colleges as accredited training, the duration of any part time senior registrar training need not be strictly prorated and allowance

can be made for commitment to the specialty and use of non-sessional time for continued study.

● Remember, too, that if you move to another region during your period of flexible training, the manpower approval moves with you. However, the educational approval and funding need to be negotiated.

● Do not give up. Remember that you have gained a great deal of knowledge and experience in workforce issues and the working of the region. This is excellent firsthand management training for your future consultant post!

With ever-increasing numbers of women graduating from medical schools, we hope that facilities for part time training will be incorporated into all training rotations and that there will be greater recognition of the validity of part time training and support for the national scheme fostered by the higher training committees and royal colleges. Virginia Bottomley in her letter to regional chairpersons pointed out:

> The joint working party on women doctors and their careers reported in January 1991 and found that part time candidates for senior registrar training are of high quality. They have well founded individual reasons for wishing to use the part time option in training for consultant posts and are a major resource and asset and a long term investment for the NHS whch cannot be wasted.

1 Bolton-Maggs P, Van Somerson V. The need for part-time work: a survey of doctors 10 years after graduation. *Br J Hosp Med* 1988; **39**: 413–16.
2 Warren V J, Wakeford R E. "We'd like to have a family"—young women doctors' opinions of maternity leave and part time training. *J R Soc Med* 1989; **82**: 528–31.
3 Allen I. *Doctors and their careers*. London: Policy Studies Institute, Blackmore Press, 1991.
4 Proctor S. Hard times—hard choices; positive decision-making for part-time women doctors. *Med Educ* 1987; **21**: 260–4.
5 Gath A. Part-time senior registrar training in child and adolescent psychiatry. *Bulletin of the Royal College of Psychiatrists* 1988; **12**: 368–9.
6 Department of Health and Social Security. Personnel Memorandum, 1979.

26 Be a general practitioner locum

David Allen Stocks

"Our senior partner has collapsed. Can you take over, starting this evening?" Jobs are rarely arranged at such short notice, but when a doctor becomes "established" as a general practitioner locum the phone never stops ringing. Always keep a diary or calendar by the phone and pencil in the dates there and then. Have nothing to do with scraps of paper or the backs of envelopes: they float away into drawers and dustbins with important information lost for ever. Double booking is the cardinal sin.

Becoming known

How does word get round that you are available for work? Try these methods:

(1) Write to local general practitioners. I suggest sending a formal letter giving the dates when you are free. Enclose a copy of your curriculum vitae. A job might not be forthcoming but general practitioners like to have a pool of locums to draw from.

(2) Write to your family health services authority. Family health services authorities are not locum agencies, but they occasionally need a locum when a singlehanded doctor is ill. The family health services authority may offer to send, for a fee, a copy of your curriculum vitae to each of the practices in its area.

(3) Circulate at postgraduate meetings. Bump into your trainer, general practice tutors, and former colleagues. This all helps to hang your name on the grapevine.

(4) Enrol with agencies (but read the small print). Local offices might be better than nationwide agencies. A doctor I know was asked to travel over 100 miles to do one afternoon's surgery. The BMA locum agency, administered from its regional offices, is free to members.

(5) Advertise in medical journals. Give some flavour to your advertisement without sounding eccentric. Market yourself as a reliable and steady worker, neither bland nor spicy.

When responding to advertisements you must be quick off the mark: vacancies are soon filled.

The interview

Interviews are usually informal. They are thought of as introductions "to meet the other partners" or "to look round the health centre". The chit-chat over coffee may be charming but don't be wrongfooted into thinking the interview is a social call. You should be armed with your current certificates and copies of your curriculum vitae.

I am usually accepted at face value. My references have never been taken up, but it would be businesslike to ask your referees beforehand if they would mind giving your reference over the phone. Be sure of your dates before the interview. If you say "Yes, I'll definitely come" when offered the job, then consider yourself caught: only illness or bereavement would let you comfortably off the hook.

Sort out pay and hours of work. You could accept the BMA guidelines on pay or use them as a basis for negotiation. There are standard rates for (a) a two-hour surgery, (b) a surgery and calls, and (c) a full day. These are self explanatory, but if night or weekend work is required, then make sure you know exactly what is expected. Also ask if the practice has any prescribing policies, such as antibiotics for sore throats. Try to comply with such policies without being a cipher. Ask for a timetable of your duties if the job lasts for longer than a day.

Before starting

When replacing a singlehanded doctor, phone the day before starting and ask about any seriously ill patients. I once called to see a

167

patient without knowing that she was dying. The breezy tone of my visit was just wrong from the start. The patient looked disappointed. Her husband did not say much, but his expression seemed to say, "Our old doctor has left us in the lurch and sent this amateur instead". The quickest glance at the notes is better than nothing.

You will need drugs for emergency use and a bag for your equipment. You will have to pay for the drugs yourself, but they can be bought in small quantities from a pharmacist. Although tablets are readily available, drugs for injection are not always in stock; the pharmacist may need a day's notice to order them from the wholesale supplier. Controlled drugs are best kept in your pocket or bag and not in your car boot. A record of these drugs should be kept as they are bought and used.

If you intend to be a locum regularly, then it is worth buying a doctor's bag rather than making do with your battered old briefcase. Do pay attention to your appearance and "image"—patients like to size up the locum, so don't look like a ragbag even though you feel like a stopgap.

Your first day

Arrive five or ten minutes early and ask to be shown round. Introduce yourself to the receptionists and the practice nurse. Ask for your name to be put on the door and find out where the doctor has gone on holiday—you will be asked this several times each surgery. Feel free to rearrange the furniture: I hate to use the desk as a defensive barrier. Find out if you shout or buzz for the first patient. If the corridor is not too long I like to go and collect each patient, although some regular attenders, primed for the buzzer, are unnerved by this little courtesy. Later in the day call in at the local pharmacy to introduce yourself.

Medical practice

As a locum I suffer from four temptations:

(1) Superficiality. Patients who want to unburden an emotional problem will mostly prefer to consult a doctor they know. My locum work is biased towards acute minor illnesses. The temptation is to be superficial—to concentrate on the disease rather than the patient. This might suit most, but you should be alert to those patients with

more deep-rooted problems. When seeing a new doctor these patients often test the water first with a minor ailment before plunging in with an emotional disclosure.

(2) Passing the buck. Not knowing the patients, you can easily fall behind appointment times, especially when these are at five minute intervals. I am then tempted to pass the buck: "Just take a few more of your tablets; they'll keep you going until your doctor comes back next week." You should do justice to the patient whose problem cannot be put off. Procrastination is a corruption of good medical practice.

(3) Showing off. It is tempting to dazzle patients with a flash of brilliant plumage, and indeed a little knowledge can be finely dressed. But then the locum flies off, leaving the nest badly disturbed for the returning doctor. This particularly applies to those "heartsink"[1] and difficult[2] patients who flatter you at their own doctor's expense. Similarly, regular prescriptions should not be changed merely for the sake of elegant variation: "Still on those old tablets? I think these new ones will suit you much better". A locum should enjoy the tenancy but should leave things neat and tidy for the sitting tenant.

(4) Lazy prescribing. In most practices the receptionist fills in the whole of the repeat prescription. All the doctor has to do is sign. Beware. Resist the importunity of harassed receptionists. Insist on seeing the notes first. Double check doses; treble check warfarin.[3] Be scrupulous with your signature; if in doubt, fail safe.

Visits

For visits you will need a map, a *British National Formulary*, the phone numbers of hospitals and ambulance control, and plenty of headed notepaper and prescriptions. An experienced receptionist will put the non-urgent visits in order so that you can drive a circular tour. Ask for the patients' phone numbers to be written on the front of the notes. Inner city visits are a nightmare for the stranger: flyovers and one-way streets, underpasses, and no-parking signs all conspire against you. Never be tempted on to an urban motorway. Street signs have been pulled down and house numbers have been printed over. Don't despair. Country visits, too, have their pleasures: roads dwindle into dirt tracks, houses hide behind trees. If you are seriously lost, ring the local police. When visiting at night, ask for all the lights to be switched on and for the curtains to be left open.

Playing fair

Most surgeries last for about two hours. Locums are not paid to the minute, so keep working with a good grace if you are still busy after two and a half hours: tomorrow's surgery might last for only an hour and forty minutes.

All the general practitioners I have worked for have been honourable employers, but watch out for a nominal one-hour surgery, paid at half of the two-hour rate, that regularly lasts all morning.

A sharp practice is to find yourself replacing two doctors. If you are overwhelmed with work, speak to the senior partner or the practice manager. Do this before cracking up.

Write in the notes as carefully as possible. Abandon your darling shorthand and stick to standard abbreviations. Write legibly or not at all—the medical secretary is a suitable judge.

If the doctor you are replacing refers patients to a particular consultant in each specialty, then try to follow suit.

One or two patients will ask for a second opinion from you. A niggling dissatisfaction with their doctor is often apparent. The patient's interests come first, of course, so the symptoms and signs must be assessed impartially, but it is unprofessional to erode any further the patient's confidence in the doctor. I believe that polite neutrality is the best response when patients criticise their doctor. Listening carefully to the patient might be enough to soothe the irritation.[4]

Frustrations and rewards

A few patients will be disappointed about not seeing their usual doctor. The hurt tone of "Where's *the* doctor?" says it all. Don't be discouraged. One day patients might become as loyal to you. Occasionally a patient will refuse to be examined. I used to be upset by this, but now I simply ask the patient to return either the following day or within a week. If the symptoms sound serious, then leave a note for the doctor when you leave.

Not being able to follow up patients is frustrating, especially when you suspect some unusual disease. I sometimes call in several weeks after leaving a surgery to inquire about such patients.

Locum general practice is ideal work for a doctor looking for a permanent job as a general practitioner. One picks up so many ideas for the perfect practice, including things to avoid. Practices are like the suburbs of London: some are up and coming, some are fashionable, and some have seen better days. Surgery accommodation varies from the palatial to the poky. But patients everywhere deserve the best. There is satisfaction in trying to practise a high standard of medicine for every patient irrespective of surroundings.

1 O'Dowd T C. Five years of heartsink patients in general practice. *BMJ* 1988; **297**: 528–30.
2 Gerrard T J, Riddell J D. Difficult patients: black holes and secrets. *BMJ* 1988; **297**: 530–2.
3 Medical Defence Union. *Annual report*. London: MDU, 1988; 40.
4 Calnan J. *Talking with patients*. London: Heinemann, 1983.

27 Job share a consultant post

Graham Thornicroft, Geraldine Strathdee

Job sharing in medicine is still a rarity, although the NHS is now beginning to make it easier. We successfully applied together for a single consultant post in community psychiatry and we describe here our experiences of how job sharing a consultant post can be made to work. Our reasons for job sharing were different: one of us has interests in community clinical service development and wanted to retain formal training links with the London School of Economics and the Open University, and the other wanted to combine clinical work with research interests in mental health service evaluation and psychiatric epidemiology.

Defining job sharing

Job sharing is an arrangement "whereby two people voluntarily share the responsibility of one full-time position. The salary and benefits are shared between them according to the time they work, and each holds a permanent part-time post".[1] It differs from part-time work, which is not shared; joint appointments, in which more than one post is shared; and job splitting, where an existing full-time post is split specifically to make work available to more people.

During the past 15 years job-sharing arrangements have become much more common. Within the NHS 92 health authorities and boards throughout England, Scotland, and Northern Ireland employ job sharers. Hospital medical posts are shared at every level of seniority, including the consultant grade, in the following special-

---

Advantages of job sharing to employers

• Job sharers' previous work experience is often complementary, and they bring to a single post a wider range of skills and experience than could an individual.[3]

• Job sharers are able to sustain a higher level of commitment and productivity in the longer term than can one employee, and in some cases staff turnover is reduced.[4]

• The arrangement increases flexibility: post holders can often cover for each other during leave without having to rely on cover provided by other colleagues, as is usually the case with full-time post holders.[5]

• In practice the job sharers often work far more than their allotted sessions and together contribute considerably more than one person in post.[6]

---

ties: psychiatry, obstetrics and gynaecology, anaesthetics, radiology, and paediatrics. Many general practitioners job share, and the BMA runs a partnership scheme to match sharers.

Job-sharing arrangements are also operating successfully for nurses, occupational therapists, pharmacists, medical social workers, and psychologists in the NHS.[2] Indeed, the post of chief executive of the Lambeth, Southwark, and Lewisham Family Health Services Authority is held on a job-sharing basis. Other public services are now well ahead of the NHS: in local government there are over 2000 job-sharing employees, and more than a third of local authorities have such arrangements.

Effect on employers

Although employing authorities are often initially cautious, job sharing offers considerable general advantages to them: there is reduced staff turnover and absenteeism, increased staff flexibility, increased productivity, greater continuity, and enhanced availability of skills. Organisations as diverse as the Stock Exchange and the Equal Opportunities Commission have conducted studies of job sharing. Their findings agree (see box).

The main concerns often voiced by employers about job-sharing arrangements are poor communication, greater overhead costs, and clinical responsibility.

173

Poor communications

Although in some specialties, such as anaesthetics, sessions may be split with little need for handover, more often good communication and clearly defined responsibilities are vital. In practice this rarely causes problems. Evaluations of job sharers invariably find that they establish regular handover sessions to ensure continuity in discharging their responsibilities.[7]

Greater overhead costs

There may be small extra costs, especially initially, in the administration of contracts, salaries, and in office space and equipment. Despite this, the head of personnel at the Stock Exchange found no significant increase in total costs of employing job sharers. Similarly, national insurance contributions for two job sharers are in almost every case less than for one post holder.[8]

Clinical responsibility

If a single caseload is shared or if job sharers each have a caseload and cross cover, an explicit arrangement is needed concerning exactly which job-sharing partner has clinical responsibility for which patients at each time during the week. This arrangement and any changes to it should be communicated to all relevant colleagues. In our case we also made sure that we would be available to colleagues by carrying a radio pager while on duty.

Practical arrangements

Since job sharing is still uncommon for doctors, potential job sharers need to be specially careful and thorough when applying for a job. To be shortlisted, applicants may need to add to the standard form their own appendixes setting out what job sharing is, its advantages to employers as well as employees, and expected clinical arrangements—for example, how continuity of care and on call rotas will be organised. We decided that we would need to convince our potential employers that we were each appointable before our joint application would be considered, and so we arranged separate pre-interview meetings. We were not told whether we would be interviewed separately or together, and so we prepared for both; the panel in fact did both.

In our clinical work we have each taken clinical responsibility for half of the caseload of the whole post and we work with separate multidisciplinary teams. We cover for each other for those sessions when the other is not on duty. We negotiated six sessions each on our appointment and the twelfth session is used as a regular planning and handover meeting to discuss clinical, research, teaching, service planning, and administrative issues.

Our usual working arrangement is that all regular clinical activities are carried out by the team's consultant. When one consultant is not on duty the job sharer becomes the responsible medical officer. During any periods when both job sharers are not available— for example, because of leave or exceptional circumstances—the clinical responsibility is taken by another colleague at the hospital. We normally cover for each other during annual leave, but we made sure in our contract that we were not obliged to cover for each other because we both have children and might need to arrange leave during school holidays.

Terms and conditions of employment

In our hospital there was no precedent for doctors to job share and so we put forward a draft set of contractual terms and conditions as the basis for negotiation with our personnel department. The main issues that we had to clarify were annual leave; allowances for sickness, study, and training leave; and car and pension entitlements. We each received a separate contract with job sharer in the title, which included the following section: "The conditions which apply to full-time employees apply to job sharers jointly (Employment Protection (Consolidation) Act, 1978). Entitlements for which employees qualify by length of service are calculated individually, and where appropriate, on a proportional basis according to the number of hours worked. The concept of proportionality is applied to the conditions of service unless otherwise specified."

We used the principle of proportionality for most of these entitlements—for example, annual leave and pension entitlements were divided pro rata to give us each 6/11 of the full allowance. However, after taking advice we stipulated that sick leave would relate to length of service and that we would be included in the statutory sick pay scheme with seven days a week each as the qualifying days.

We requested and received a full entitlement each for training and

175

study leave and car allowance. We argued that to be effective in our posts we could not accept going on half a training course each and that half a travel allowance was not efficient because our post was to develop community-oriented mental health services. The essential user's payment is made on an individual basis to each job sharer, with milage reimbursement at the same rate as for full-time essential users.

The arrangement for our pay was straightforward: we receive the same rates as full-time staff and are paid according to the number of hours worked; we are each graded at the appropriate level in the incremental scale (one of us had worked previously as a consultant). We included in the contract that continuous service entitlements would apply for previous periods of service within the NHS and related research organisations. Similarly, pension entitlements were rated according to hours worked on the same basis as full-time employees and previous qualifying service was recognised for calculating payments. We were also advised that full merit awards were payable if at least six sessions were worked. In negotiating our contract we were greatly helped by the organisation New Ways to Work, which we strongly recommend to potential job sharers.[1]

If one job sharer leaves

The most difficult issue in discussing the terms of the contract was the arrangement in case one of us left the shared post. Our managers needed to ensure that the service would continue fully staffed and that they retained a degree of flexibility in using consultant expertise for the development of the whole service. On our side we needed to maintain job security and to guard against the future possibility of being paired with an unsuitable partner. People considering sharing a post should give this issue detailed thought and come to a clear written agreement with their employing authority.

In our case we agreed that should one partner leave, the employer would first offer that portion of the post to the remaining partner. If this was not accepted, the unfilled post would be advertised as a job-share vacancy by the health authority and the incumbent would be fully included in the selection procedure. If no suitable candidate was appointed the post would be advertised full time and the remaining post holder would be protected under the terms of the employing authority's redeployment procedure.

In post

Our main difficulties came in putting together a strong case when we applied jointly for a single post. Just after our appointment some colleagues expressed confusion and even amusement about what was for them a novel working arrangement: we were asked about our "job-splitting" or "work-sharing" scheme. Although we have continued to mention that we are each half time, the formal arrangement was soon forgotten and one of the big practical disadvantages of job sharing is the expectation from colleagues that each partner should take on the non-clinical duties of a full-time post holder. We have both been invited to participate in increasing numbers of committees, teaching sessions, planning groups, and audit meetings, and stating that we are each half time has sometimes met with short shrift. We started job sharing as friends and this has been an enormous advantage in making the arrangement work well: we find it hard to imagine sharing a post unless there is at least mutual trust and respect.

Within the remainder of the public sector, in private industry, and more recently in other NHS disciplines, more adaptable working arrangements are now increasingly well established. Medicine is anachronistic in limiting all but full-time appointments and in excluding other more imaginative options such as paternity leave, work exchanges, and career breaks.[9, 10] The NHS now needs to combine high standards of treatment and care with working conditions that will give more control, flexibility, and job satisfaction to its staff.

Acknowledgements

We thank New Ways to Work, Sue Osborne, and Sue Williams (job sharing chief executive at Lambeth, Southwark, and Lewisham Family Health Services Authority) for clear and helpful information, and our managers, Eric Byers and Jeremy Christie-Brown, for creative support.

1 Equal Opportunities Commission. *Job sharing: improving the quality and availability of part-time work*. London: EOC, 1981.
2 Lempp H, Heslop A. Pioneering spirit. *Senior Nurse* 1987; 7: 24–6.
3 New Ways to Work. *Job sharing: putting policy into practice*. London: New Ways to Work, 1987.
4 New Ways to Work. *Job sharing in the health service*. London: New Ways to Work, 1989.
5 Walton P. *Job sharing: a practical guide*. London: Kogan Page, 1990.

6 Meager N, Buchan J, Rees C. *Job sharing in the National Health Service*. London: Institute of Manpower Studies, 1989. (Report No 174)
7 Industrial Relations Services. Job sharing survey. *Employment Trends* 1989; **6**: 441.
8 Boyle A. *Job sharing: a study of the costs, benefits and employment rights of job sharers*. London: Equal Opportunities Commission, 1980.
9 Allen I. *Any room at the top? A study of doctors and their careers*. London: Policy Studies Institute, 1988.
10 Bolton-Maggs P, Van Someren V, Lefford F. The need for part-time work: a survey of doctors 10 years after graduation. *Br J Hosp Med* 1988; **5**: 413–16.

28 Start in private practice

Anthony E Young

I suspect that most senior registrars are appointed to consultant posts in the NHS with only the sketchiest of notions about private practice. This may be an encouraging reflection on their commitment to the principles of the NHS but it leaves them unprepared for private practice, and the best advice I can give for the newly appointed consultant wishing to enter this is that he should find an approachable senior colleague and unashamedly ask for advice about the practicalities and local arrangements. I was fortunate enough to have colleagues who gave me this advice unbidden, but for those of you too shy to make that approach the following broad observations are made. They are based on experiences in surgical practice in London and I accept that they may not be relevant to the practice of venereology in Wick or anaesthesia in Penzance.

Why private practice?

From the patient's point of view private practice entails the buying of a consultant's time. In addition, the patient is expecting to buy comfort and convenience. Sadly, many patients believe that they can buy a "better" consultant opinion or a more effective operation privately and, though I would like to believe that there is no difference in the opinions and skills available in the two different settings, I must ruefully admit that the current fraught and constricted practice in the NHS may mean that better medicine is indeed available in the private sector, even when the same doctor is concerned.

179

Overall, time is probably the most important factor, and after a few relaxed half to one hour new patient consultations you will quickly wonder how we do justice to patients and their diseases in the hectic NHS schedule. Adequate time is a pleasure as well as a necessity; it improves your clinical habits and sets standards that you should hope to be able to emulate in the NHS. Much has been written about the relationship between the NHS and private practice and it is not the purpose of this chapter to root around in the ideological detritus of the various arguments. For the moment the two exist in parallel, and consultants overlap between them. The consultant's task is to make the system work to the benefit of all patients and there is no reason why proper care of NHS patients and of private patients should be incompatible if consultants use their skills honestly and their time effectively.

It goes without saying that the private patient expects the consistent personal attention of one doctor, but it is a sad indication of people's perception of the uncertainties of the NHS that they will often ask at a private consultation, "And will *you* be doing the operation?"

Setting aside the time

Even very busy consultants' NHS commitments will leave some free time for private practice. If they are less than full time that extra time will be complete sessions; if they are truly full time, the consultants may need to find that time at the beginning or end of the working day or at weekends. Wherever that time is found, it is best to structure it. Arrange a definite time of the week to see patients and if you are a surgeon arrange a regular operating time. Without that, not only is your orderly practice disrupted, but life becomes difficult for your secretary and your family. Don't be coy about these sessions: they are a perfectly proper part of your professional life and should feature on your hospital timetable just as your hospital schedule appears on your private timetable. There is nothing more infuriating for NHS staff than a consultant who unpredictably dematerialises and cannot be contacted.

A particular problem for those who practice in London is grappling with the tight schedules required in the treatment of patients from overseas, who frequently come unannounced and want their definitive treatment today or tomorrow (or even yesterday). All you can do is fit things in as quickly as possible, at the same time exhorting them and their advisers to give some warning next time.

Private practice is, in essence, singlehanded practice: the patient is paying for you, not someone else. This potentially makes the taking of time for holidays and meetings difficult, and shows how important it is to have an effective partnership or cross cover with your colleagues for those occasions. Partnerships also allow you to offer a comprehensive emergency service, something that is not widespread in the private sector.

Premises and secretaries

Private practice must be organised from some geographically fixed base. Traditionally this is the consultant's "rooms", the place where the secretary can be found and where patients are seen. Increasingly, consultants see patients in several places, perhaps at home and also in private hospitals. That is all very well and it may increase the options for the patients, but for the colleagues who refer and for the patient on the telephone a central point of contact is vital. Even for those with a secretary, an answering machine and probably a fax on a separate line are crucial.

Few can now afford rooms and a secretary for their sole use. A joint practice—or sessional arrangements in a private clinic—is substantially cheaper and almost as satisfactory. Wherever you practice, it is worth remembering that comfort and convenience are not just the private hospital's concern. Your consulting room should be pleasant and tranquil to be in, for the benefit of both you and your patient. Choose your secretary carefully; she or he too should be pleasant and tranquil, sympathetic on the telephone, and endlessly patient with the disruptions that will occur.

Full timers and those with small private practices may use their NHS secretaries but this is open to abuse, and the rules, remuneration, and hours need to be set very carefully at the outset and the agreement of the hospital administration obtained.

Many consultants employ their spouses as their private secretaries and receptionists. A spouse's salary is tax deductible under schedule D, but to be so must actually be paid to him or her.

A fair amount of paper flutters around every consultation: notes have to be made up, addresses taken, tests and admissions arranged, bills sent. This inevitable mini bureaucracy works more smoothly if the secretary is in the same place as the consultation. If you are of the right bent, a microcomputer might well ease these chores, and there are specific software packages available for this.

For London readers I should perhaps add a note here about Harley Street. Indeed, not just for London readers. Otherwise sane people travel miles from hospitals in the outer suburbs to get to an address in Harley Street, where they see patients who have made the same awful journey. I wonder for whose benefit this time-honoured quirk persists. In fairness, however, I should admit that Harley Street and its environs contain a very talented and comprehensive set of medical facilities—though nobody should be under the illusion that the address guarantees quality, as any reader of the Sunday newspapers will know. The phenomenon of Harley Street persists out of conservatism and snobbery as much as for any other reason and I don't think that new consultants really ought to feel an obligation to take rooms or sessions there, certainly not at the outset of their careers, unless the romance of the Harley Street reputation really appeals to them.

Where to practise

Private patients still have the option of either a private bed in an NHS hospital or a bed in a private hospital. Hospitals in the NHS may lack the thick carpets and warm lighting of the private clinics, but make up with a wider range of medical services. Where you admit patients depends on their wishes and their diseases. Not all private hospitals can cope with complex or severe illness, and in dealing with these the full NHS team has advantages. Remember, however, that though such patients may be educational, junior NHS staff may resent time spent with them, and their efforts should not be taken for granted or abused. You should also consult the *Handbook on Management of Private Practice in Health Service Hospitals in England and Wales*, available from the Department of Health.

When a surgeon has another doctor to assist him or her at a private operation in a private hospital the assistant must be paid—and promptly. Some surgeons do not pay if the patient defaults; though this may serve as an object lesson in financial reality, it seems to me to be improper. When the assistant is the patient's general practitioner, a fee is usually still expected, though the amount may be difficult to judge.

Private hospitals are, in general, pleasant places in which to practise, and nurses are less stressed than they seem to be in the NHS. The quieter environment and the smaller scale of most such hospitals give them an atmosphere reminiscent of cottage hospitals of old.

Developing a practice

Britain's position near the bottom of the European "league table" of doctors per head of population guarantees that in the NHS none of us sit in the outpatient clinic twiddling our thumbs waiting for patients to be referred. One is led to believe that in certain well-heeled southern country towns the same applies in private practice, but for most consultants there is the sobering realisation that in the private sector practice has to be earned, not taken for granted. This is one of the virtues of the activity. Advertising for practice is not allowed beyond a restrained card to general practitioners and colleagues advising them that you are available and giving them your address and your consultation times; after that, like the owner of the newly opened shop or gallery, you must just sit smiling confidently and wait to see what happens.

At the outset some patients will come, as doctors try you out; after that your practice can go either way—up or down. One would like to think that the progress of one's practice reflected the quality of service offered, but it is, of course, more complicated than that. Social contacts probably count more than anything—a fact not wasted on those who, to the disgust of their colleagues, spend time and money developing social bonds with people with whom they might not otherwise bother to pass the time of day. Nevertheless, it is nice to think that patients come because they want to see you, and there is enormous satisfaction in seeing as new patients people who come on the specific recommendation of a patient previously treated. It is worth noting in passing at this point that though it is preferable for patients to be referred from their general practitioners or other doctors, as they are in the health service, there is no rule that says this must be done, and private practice continues to offer a convenient escape route for patients who feel dissatisfied with their general practitioner or local hospital. Most health insurance companies do, however, insist on referral being from a general practitioner. Unless the patient forbids you, it is correct always to write to the general practitioner after the consultation.

There are two fallacies to beware of. First, do not expect to inherit

183

the practice of your NHS predecessor. Very few give up their NHS and private practices simultaneously. Second, never believe what you are told about the size of other people's practices, particularly if they are vulgar enough to tell you themselves. Such claims are like fishing stories, and the magnification quotient ranges upwards from two times reality.

Money

We are all spoilt by being brought up in the NHS with a regular salary and hardly a care in the world about the money we spend on our patients. For this reason the financial side of private practice brings surprises for the newcomer.

The nice surprise is, of course, the extra income that it brings. The other surprise is the sudden awareness of how much everything costs. You see the bills for the bed and the blood tests, and if the patient is uninsured you must quickly develop a lean view of what is really essential for his or her care. Those few extra days in hospital can set a patient back £1000, the computed tomography done to document the lesions that you are not going to treat £400, the frozen section done so that the nature of the lump will be known tonight not tomorrow £350. Now try pricing unnecessary parenteral nutrition, fancy drugs, the endoscopies to watch an ulcer healing, and you quickly realise how prodigal the health service can be. Uninsured or underinsured patients bring with them a lot of anxieties about the cost of their care and it is important to spell out very carefully for such people the possible costs that they are or may be committing themselves to; indeed they may need to be persuaded back into the arms of the NHS. This is allowed. Patients may change horses in midstream, but only once in any particular episode of illness. Patients very rarely ask how much their treatment will cost, and the doctor is honour bound to have done those sums even if the patient doesn't ask. One colleague of mine produces written estimates like a builder. That is no bad thing, and incidentally one does not need to add VAT: doctors are exempt.

The financial side of private practice requires two things. The first is accurate and tidy bookkeeping; the second is an accountant. New consultants who think they can manage their own accounts will, unless they take an unhealthy pleasure in figures, find themselves quickly out of their depth in the murkier corners of self-employed income tax, schedule 4 National Insurance exemption, and rolled-over capital gains tax. I doubt if many accountants inject their own haemorrhoids and likewise I would advise you not to attempt your own accounts. It is worth talking to your accountant well before the first tax demand appears, as a certain amount of forward planning is needed. You may, for instance, need to set the end of your accounting year at the end of April, allowing an extra year's breathing space before the first tax is due. To someone brought up on PAYE the need to write cheques for the Inland Revenue on fees long since spent may come as an embarrassment. Thus from the start it is prudent to set aside, say, 25% of your private earnings in anticipation of a juicy tax demand. Although schedule D is more generous with allowances than the schedule E of PAYE, the costs of setting up in practice are by no means all tax deductible, so don't rush out and buy a new car.

New consultants may be anxious about what fees they should charge patients. This need not be a source of anxiety, as in each geographical area there are fairly standard fees for new and for follow-up consultations, and the insurance companies issue lists categorising operations into minor, intermediate, major, and major-plus types. In addition, they settle the amount that they will reimburse for an operation in any category. There are ill-concealed murmurs of dissatisfaction about the levels of these fees and their unbalanced nature favouring certain specialties. Nevertheless, insured patients reasonably expect to be charged what the insurance company specifies, and if you intend to charge more than that you ought to tell the patient in advance. Although the fee guidelines of the British United Provident Association (BUPA), Private Patients Plan (PPP), and the BMA offer a welcome reference point, they have been criticised by the Monopolies and Merger's Commission. If they are banned, the business of fee setting will become vexatious to all.

Conclusion

However small it might be, most people find private practice is instructive, stimulating, and rewarding—so much so that its enticements may be considerable—and it will thus do no harm to conclude with a warning about abuses of private practice that can too easily be slipped into. These include over treating, over charging, and over valuing your own skills so that you are tempted to treat in private practice those conditions that you would refer to your colleagues in the context of the health service. Lastly, remember to be punctilious about your commitments in the NHS. Don't let an enthusiasm for private practice nibble into your NHS time. Your junior staff may not get any formal education in private practice, but watching you will be their informal education and it should be correct.

29 Work abroad

Anne Savage

In times past the decision to work in what was then generally known as "the mission field" required long thought, involving, as it did, a lifetime's service, discomfort, isolation, and not a little danger. On the other hand, continuous, interesting work was assured. The situation is now reversed, so that easy travel and communications, short contracts, safety, and reasonable comfort must be set against the formidable problems of re-establishment.

When and where

That being so, your first objective, if you contemplate spending even a short time abroad, must be to secure, as far as possible, your return. Much will depend on your status when you go, but for those already established on the specialist ladder, seek out a sympathetic consultant and discuss your plans; research the possibilities of a future job. The subject of proleptic appointments—that is, those made a year or more in advance—is under discussion, and a few exist. They certainly bring a sense of security to a troubled mind, but be warned of two possible problems: you may find it difficult, because a replacement is lacking, to return on the appointed date, and you may change your mind. If your ambitions are towards general practice, then the time spent overseas may count as part of your general professional training, but there are no rules, so approach your postgraduate dean. Keep in touch while you are away and keep a log of interesting cases. It will provide fascinating reading for your old age, and may prove useful before that as evidence of experience and ability. Do not neglect research. Third World countries are so full of unexplained problems that a reasonable project could easily be devised and carried through even in the absence of sophisticated equipment.

When to go is most often a matter of circumstance, but those in a position to choose might consider the following points. It is easier to study and pass examinations if you continue in an unbroken succession of posts. You will get more out of your time spent abroad if you are already some way up the professional ladder; this applies especially to surgeons and obstetricians. You may be able to incorporate your overseas appointment into your training programme, and while this applies mainly to general practitioners, a few specialist accredited posts exist; inquire at the appropriate royal college if in doubt. It may well be that experience of other disciplines leads to a wavering in your dedication and a move is more easily made at an earlier stage. If children are involved, their education must be considered. Up to the age of 7 the local school will serve; after that the cultural differences become sharper, and, apart from a few good international schools, the choice lies between boarding school and home tuition.

Where to go? No problem as to country because of the global shortage of doctors. Avoid South America unless you are proficient in Spanish or Portuguese. Parts of Africa are francophone, otherwise the lingua franca is English. Religion rarely causes difficulty, statements such as "strong Christian commitment required" being self-explanatory, but many mission and ex-mission hospitals, even when staffed by religious orders, accept recruits of all faiths, and none. With the acceptance of South Africa into the global family, political prohibitions have mostly disappeared, but local ones may persist. They are likely to be very local, and easily overcome by a slight geographical shift.

Consider carefully the type of hospital, often designated by the number of doctors on the establishment (not necessarily the number in post at any one time), and unless you are very self-confident and a handy general surgeon, avoid the one-doctor ones. Promises of back-up are worthless if the only road has been washed away by rain.

Paperwork

The choice made, set about getting your papers. In almost all cases a work permit and registration with the medical council are

188

necessary. Forms can be voluminous and forbidding. They are devised by public service departments with the object of sifting out the dross, of which a fair bit floats round Third World countries. Do the best you can; details of your kindergarten successes are not necessary; but do read the small print, and remember that a commissioner for oaths is not necessarily a notary public, and only the latter may certify some photocopies.

At the same time write direct to the medical superintendent or a senior doctor. Sending agencies cannot be expected to be fully up to date, and departments of health are often very vague, and sometimes positively misleading, about conditions at the periphery. It is as well, before the spouse and children step wearily into their new home, to make sure it has some furniture and means of cooking. In addition to the basic issues—housing, shops, schools and recreational facilities —make a list of the smaller things that might cause problems: voltage, refrigeration, radio reception, and availability of any regular medicines and contraceptives. Do not forget a car. Public transport is mostly overcrowded and unreliable, taxis outside the larger towns, nonexistent. A secondhand vehicle may be available, but if not, with an eye to spares, find out which make is most favoured locally.

Look forward

Between decision and departure gather as much information as you can. Medical superintendents desperate for staff can paint a rosy picture and make extravagant promises. Forewarned is forearmed, not necessarily frightened off. Contact with someone recently returned is invaluable, and students on electives, in particular, can be a source of unbiased and uninhibited comment. Extend your list to include the little things that mean a lot when you are miles from the nearest shop. Old *BMJ*s may serve as toilet paper; nothing substitutes for soap.

It is easier to settle if you know something about the country, its history and people. Hunt the libraries and consider attending a course. Some professional preparation is advisable, though it is comforting to realise that even in the tropics most of the patients will be suffering from "European" conditions. Books and audio-visual aids are helpful for those unable to attend a formal course, and informal education may be arranged in the host country. Fortify yourself against cultural deprivation by taking or arranging for a supply of cassettes and any hobby materials. Most importantly, if travelling as a pair, one of whom is not medically qualified, consider the role of the partner. It is essential that he or she is willingly involved and an active participant. Failure to work through this problem has led to contracts, sometimes the marital one, being prematurely terminated. As with so many aspects of living in developing countries, anxieties are often dispelled by reality. Particular talents and abilities are in such short supply that anyone healthy, flexible, and willing will soon be pressed into service.

Flexibility is, indeed, the most important quality to take with you. Couple it with a degree of circumspection, particularly with regard to politics. Although it is true that the major problems of the world will be solved only by political action, this is not true at the local level, where partisanship may divide, alienate, and ultimately destroy all you have attempted. You may find the local people watchful and uncommunicative at first, so learn enough of the language and customs for basic courtesy. Failure to greet formally or shake hands may be greatly, if silently, resented, whereas the reward for your slight effort will be genuine friendship. In the hospital honesty is the only policy. If you don't know something, say so. Medical cowboys, like medical tourists, are distrusted and resented, and, except in the few establishments still boasting long-serving medical superintendents, information is rarely *de haut en bas*, more an exchange between peers.

Most of the anxieties that afflict intending travellers disappear on arrival. Perhaps a few can be dispelled here. With the exception of areas of war or anarchy, you will probably be safer than in the UK, and there, as here, the main danger is from traffic accidents. Given adequate prophylaxis against the obvious hazards—malaria and so on—the incidence of disease is probably much the same, gastrointestinal replacing respiratory incidents in the rich tapestry of daily life. Do not fear being stranded; help and hospitality are universally to be found. New techniques are easier to learn when the mystique that surrounds so much British apprenticeship is dispelled. If, after sufficient time for mutual adjustment, incompatibilities persist, transfer to another hospital can usually be arranged.

Finally, in times of doubt and uncertainty, cling to two incontrovertible facts. Far more doctors working overseas stay on rather than return prematurely, and many who originally came as students or immediately after registration later return as mature doctors. In fact, your main problem may be, in more than one sense, adapting back.

190

Agencies sending doctors and other health workers to developing countries

Action Health 2000
The Gate House
25 Gwydir Street
Cambridge CB1 2LG
Telephone: 01223-301896

The British Red Cross
9 Grosvenor Crescent
London SW1X 7EJ
Telephone: 0171-235 5454
Specialists only; surgeons and anaesthetists preferred.

Christians Abroad
1 Stockwell Green
London SW9 9HP
Telephone: 0171-737 7811
Christian commitment required for overseas workers.

Church Missionary Society (CMS)
Partnership House
157 Waterloo Road
London SE1 8XN
Telephone: 0171-928 8681

Christoffel-Blindenmission
Contact: Andreas Pruisken
Overseas Personnel
Niebelungenstr 124
D-6140 Bensheim 4
Germany
Telephone: 49 62 51 13 10
Special interests: blindness and physical disablement.

International Co-operation for Development (formerly CIIR)
Unit 3
Canonbury Yard
190a New North Road
London N1 7BJ
Telephone: 0171-354 1883
Primary/community health care.

International Health Exchange
Africa Centre
38 King Street
London WC2E 8JT
Telephone: 0171-836 5833
Keeps a register of positions vacant and may be helpful in providing up-to-date addresses and telephone numbers of other agencies. Charges an annual fee on a sliding scale. Telephone for further information.

Medicins sans Frontières
3-4 St Andrews Hill
London EC4 5BY
Telephone: 0171-329 6936
Medical care for victims of disaster

Medical Aid for Palestinians (MAP)
33a Islington Park Street
London N1 1QB
Telephone: 0171-226 4114

Overseas Development Administration
Abercrombie House
Eaglesham Road
East Kilbride
Glasgow G75 8EA
Telephone: 0171-917 7000 or 01355-844000

Save the Children Fund (UK)
Overseas Personnel
17 Grove Lane
London SE5 8RD
Telephone: 0171-703 5400
Previous relevant overseas experience required.

Continued

Tear Fund
100 Church Street
Teddington
London TW11 8QE
Telephone: 0181-977 9144
Skilled personnel needed.

United Nations Association
  International Service (UNAIS)
Suite 3A
Hunter House
57 Goodramgate
York YO1 2LS
Telephone: 01904 647799

Voluntary Services Overseas
  (VSO)
317 Putney Bridge Road
London SW15 2PN
Telephone: 0181-780 2266

Voluntary Missionary
  Movement (VMM)
Comboni House
London Road
Sunningdale
Berkshire SL5 0JY
Telephone: 01344-875380

Publications

Brown H, Thomas R. *Brits abroad*. London: Express Newspapers Ltd, 1981.
Sadly, now out of print. Get a copy if you can.

Daily Telegraph Guide to Working Abroad.
London: Daily Telegraph Books, 1993.

Guardian Weekly.
A weekly digest of articles from the *Guardian, Le Monde,* and the *New York Times.* For subscription form and annual rates, contact Guardian Newspapers, 119 Farringdon Road, London EC1R 3ER; telephone: 0171-278 2332 *or* 164 Deansgate, Manchester M60 2RR; telephone: 0161-832 7200.

Courses

Centre for International Briefing
Farnham Castle
Farnham
Surrey
Telephone: 01252-721197
Four-day briefings.

International Health Exchange has a series of courses. Please ring for details.

VMM Runs two courses a year, each lasting five to six weeks.

30 Visit a health centre in a developing country

P A G Gibson, A McClelland

Most people in the world will not see a doctor when they are sick. Their nearest health worker will be a primary health care worker based in a village, aid post, or health centre. These health workers at the periphery of the health care system experience major problems of lack of supervision, leadership, supplies, and support. It is increasingly realised that training workers and posting them to rural health centres is not enough to ensure delivery of the quality and quantity of health care required to reach the goal of health for all by the year 2000. To reach this goal these workers require appropriate supervision.

Supervision has been defined as the overall range of measures to ensure that personnel carry out their activities effectively and become more competent at their work. The supervision of health centres is often best provided by district medical officers based in hospitals. As an important part of this process is visiting the peripheral health workers we will describe some points that a medical officer needs to bear in mind when planning and making a visit to a health centre. This protocol will need adjustment to suit local conditions and could be modified for use by, for example, a visiting pharmacist or specialist obstetrician.

Communication

Good communication is very important for the optimum functioning of any health system. All means available should be used to increase the quality and quantity of communication in primary

---

Main components of a health centre visit

- Good communication with all health workers
- Teaching and discussion
- Seeing patients with health workers
- Tour of health centre
- Assessing performance
- Follow up and feedback to health centre

---

health care—for example, radio, telephone, correspondence (reports, newsletters, feedback on referred patients), and ambulance or vehicle connections. A visit is an opportunity for the highest quality communication—and there is no substitute for it. The more regular and frequent that visits can be, the better. If possible, visits should be arranged for different days so as to include different aspects of health centre work: antenatal clinic, well baby clinic, tuberculosis and leprosy clinic, village patrol, aid post visit, and community health meeting. The best arrangement is if the same person can make repeated visits and build up a good relationship with the staff.

Once the time and date of the visit have been decided it is very important to keep to it, whether it is a visit every second Thursday of the month or once every six months. The ever-demanding hospital workload must not be allowed to interfere with the important but hidden needs and workloads in the community. If the visits are more than two months apart it is worth writing to give advance notice and to confirm nearer the time by telephone, radio, or post. Everyone is wrong footed when a doctor arrives unexpectedly, tired and thirsty after a gruelling three-hour trip in a bumpy vehicle.

As important as good communication is the visitor's general attitude. It should not be that of a critical external inspector but that of a member of the same health team, or a friend, coming to work together constructively to improve health care. It helps to try to create the concept of "our health centre and hospital" rather than "your health centre and my hospital". Team building and friendship are helped along by learning everyone's names and simply remembering to say "good morning" and "thank you". Always try to have tea break together; better still, stay for a midday or evening meal. Do not rush back to base and skimp on this—it will strengthen the

Teaching and discussion: common problems should be emphasised

- Child health
  cough
  diarrhoea
  immunisation
  fever
  convulsions
  nutrition
- Maternal health
  antenatal care
  birth control
  management of labour
- Communicable diseases
  water supply
  waste disposal
  tuberculosis
  malaria
  leprosy
- Sexually transmitted diseases (including HIV)
- Revision of previous teaching sessions

team, and conversation will often produce revelations and insights that would otherwise be missed. This is always a good time to promote good communication within the health centre—for example, by the use of a notice board and encouraging weekly informal meetings of the staff of the health centre. Communication between the health centre and its subcentres, dispensaries, villages, and communities is important and needs to be encouraged.

Teaching

Teaching and discussion often follow on from general conversation at tea break. Never come away from a visit without leaving behind some of your knowledge and skills, but resist requests to give a short lecture. Lectures are a passive exercise for the audience and not very effective. It is much better with a small group to stimulate a tutorial type discussion and facilitate contributions from everyone. It often helps to bring along a few prepared questions or pictures to get the ball rolling. Ask people for their solutions to problems. Base

195

your teaching on common problems and use established protocols, standard treatments, and standard texts wherever possible.

Fostering the concept of a health team and the provision of continuing education can be promoted further by a staff exchange between the health centre and the hospital for a few weeks each year.

Seeing patients

Seeing patients with the health centre staff reveals many of the daily problems of providing care in the front line, and it also gives an opportunity to watch people actually dealing with patients. Often, particular inpatients and outpatients will be referred to the doctor. Always strive to manage them using established protocols and standard treatments. You will be closely watched, and you will be assessed just as critically as you will assess the health centre workers. This opportunity for teaching on patients should be taken. Do not confine yourself to those referred cases, but also review the other inpatients and maternity cases. It is beneficial to sit alongside staff and see routine patients as they present to the outpatient clinics. Show the staff how you manage cases of "my baby is coughing", plot children's weights in health books, give nutrition advice, and examine women who come to the centre for antenatal care. Health workers are impressed if you can roll up your sleeves and join in. Often there will be staff and their children to see. Usually they are not very sick, so guard against giving them unnecessary treatment but do give them plenty of time and attention.

Tour of the health centre

Do not march around the health centre with a clipboard checking off items on a report sheet. You are there to encourage and improve, not pass or fail. It is important to have a checklist but best to commit it to memory while travelling to the health centre and to leave the clipboard in your bag until writing your report. Improvements will take time to happen, but with encouragement and regular reviews they will occur.

It is important not to forget to check basics such as the water supply and the disposal of waste. The management of diarrhoeal illnesses is substandard if a health centre does not have good toilet and washing facilities; if we ensure supplies of single-use needles for injection but these are then discarded into wastepaper bins, the

Tour of health centre

- Ground and buildings
- Water supply
- Dispensary
- Cold chain
- Steriliser
- Nutrition garden
- Waste disposal
    toilets
    dressings
    placentas
    needles
- Maternity equipment
    light for night time and suturing
    blood pressure equipment
    stethoscope
    fetal stethoscope
    delivery pack
    intravenous fluids
- Child health
    weighing scales
    auroscope
    thermometer
    Road to Health books

gardener and cleaner remain at risk. Maintaining a good dispensary and cold chain are difficult, and time should be spent helping with these two tasks.

Assessing performance

Assessment of performance is not a question of pass or fail but an indication of present performance and a means of identifying priorities and areas for improvement. Assessment is made all the time during teaching, discussion, seeing patients, and touring the health centre. Comprehensive checklists can be devised to assist with assessing clinical skills, dispensary, quality of health education activities, and other functions.

Health centres are usually expected to collect and submit to headquarters large amounts of data and statistics. This activity can

197

come to be a health centre's number one priority and consume vast amounts of time, to the detriment of providing patient services. The data often include notification of births, deaths, and notifiable diseases and reports of the number of clinic attendances and number of immunisations given. Rather than simply being swallowed up by a distant bureaucracy the data can be used locally to provide simple and quick feedback of the health centre's performance. Monthly bar charts are easily constructed to show, for example, monthly deliveries, perinatal mortality, and notification of infectious diseases. Immunisation rates can be plotted and compared with an uptake of, for example, 80% of an estimate of the target population. These activities are instructive, and staff enjoy plotting on a map geographical data such as the place of residence of typhoid cases. Assessing performance can be enjoyable.

Follow up and feedback

As the time for departure approaches it is important to state what actions you intend taking when you return to base. Problems will have been identified during the visit—for example, drug shortages, missing or broken equipment, or the need for reports, guidelines, and books. State clearly what you will do, and take these actions promptly. Previous reports should be read before going on a visit to ensure that actions have been taken. Recording a visit and writing a report may be a chore, but this is important. Document performance so that change can be appreciated.

A report may be a page in a book or a structured report form used in your district. The advantages of using a structured report are that it serves as a checklist; all visitors and supervisors use the same format; and copies are easily retained to monitor progress over months and years. Copies of reports should be supplied to the health centre, and one copy should be posted on the centre's notice board.

Often the return trip is more crowded than the outward trip. There may be patients to transfer, samples to carry, staff hitching a ride, and a gift of fruit. Such visits are the highlights of working in health care in a district, both for doctors making the visits and for health centre staff receiving them. Doctors can reach out to many more people through primary health care in this way than by staying tied to their hospitals. The surprise is always how well the hospital coped in the doctor's absence.

Further reading

Flahault D, Piot M, Franklin A. *The supervision of health personnel at district level.* Geneva: WHO, 1988.

Larsen J V. Supervision of peripheral obstetric units. *Trop Doc* 1987; **17**: 77–81.

McMahon R, Barton E, Piot M. *On being in charge: a guide for middle-level management in primary health care.* Geneva: WHO, 1980.

Amonoo-Lartson R, Ebrahim G J, Lovel H J, Ranken J P. *District health care: challenges for planning, organisation and evaluation in developing countries.* London: Macmillan, 1984.

Werner D, Bower B. *Helping health workers learn.* Palo Alto, California: Hesperian Foundation, 1982.

King M, King F, Martodipoero S. *Primary child care: a manual for health workers.* Oxford: Oxford University Press, 1978.

31 Take a sabbatical from general practice

Ian Tait

The secret of success in achieving a sabbatical from general practice is sufficient motivation. There will always be difficulties to overcome, and a momentum needs to be maintained if the bags are really to get packed, the farewells said, the dog found a home and the front door finally closed. Motivation can be entirely self-generated, but it helps a lot if others share your commitment. The people you really have to win over are, first and foremost, yourself, then your family, and then your practice partners. Once this is done, there will be other practical difficulties but none of these is likely to prevent you, although they may annoy and delay you.

Convincing yourself

Why take a sabbatical? I think there are overwhelming reasons why doctors working in general practice should have a sabbatical period away from their practices. General practice is for most of us a long-service affair. In the early years we have a lot to stimulate and challenge us; we have to settle into our practice and build it as near to our heart's desire as we can, and come to terms with the inevitable compromises. After that there is often little outward change to provoke a fresh surge of interest and energy. The "burn out" syndrome is now recognised as a real problem in the middle and late years of a practitioner's medical career. When it happens, most soldier on but it can be a disenchanting business and leads all too easily to apathetic time serving, which is bad for the doctor, the practice and, of course, the patients. Some doctors take to alcohol,

200

others to love affairs, but a safer remedy is to take sabbatical leave. Unfortunately, it is often those most in need of this who are least able to organise it. I believe appropriate sabbaticals should be thought of not as an optional extra, but as a necessary part of our professional lives—just as it is in university departments, and for the same reason of course.

The recent changes in the organisation of general practice seem to have increased the sense of pressure felt by many doctors, and also the feeling that their ability to respond creatively to new challenges is being frustrated by a burdensome bureaucracy. In theory, of course, many of the changes were intended to stimulate initiative and variation. There are such opportunities, but they require new ideas and a fresh enthusiasm if they are to be taken. An appropriate sabbatical could be just what is needed to provide new thinking, new skills, and new energy.

The doctor's family

More plans for taking a sabbatical come to grief because of the disruption it threatens to cause to the lives of other members of the family than for any other reason. There needs to be a lot of honest communication and a willingness to compromise. Above all, don't take the agreement of your family for granted. Sabbaticals work best if they are seen as offering something for everyone.

Convincing the practice

If we really believe, as I think we should, that a sabbatical period is an important part of our professional life, then it should be discussed and agreed in principle as a practice policy. This should happen long before there are specific plans for any particular individual to take sabbatical leave. At any given time in a practice there is always going to be at least one partner who feels stretched for cash and will veto any sudden, unexpected, and unagreed practice expense. Appropriate support and funding for a partner to take sabbatical leave cannot be generated on the instant. Some practices write sabbatical arrangements into their practice agreement together with long-term plans for funding. It would be good if this became the rule rather than the exception. Matters that need to be covered in such agreements include: when partners are entitled to take leave and for how long; how the practice work is to be covered, including

201

the employment and appointment of locums, and the finances involved. The responsibility for the efficient running of the practice in the absence of doctors taking sabbatical leave should fall on the practice. The departing doctor will have more than enough to do.

Financial aspects

The question of the expense of locum cover is likely to be the single most important factor in deciding what you do with your sabbatical. If you are going to be personally responsible for the cost of providing a locum, you will probably need to take paid work. This can turn out to be something of a busman's holiday. Traditionally, the idea of a sabbatical does include a sense of unpressurised time, and a chance to stand back and take stock. We should try to preserve this ideal. Financial support can come from a number of sources. The safest is some pre-planned arrangement within the practice. If this is not available, the next most obvious step is to apply for prolonged study leave.

Department of Health prolonged study leave (3–12 months)

Details of the prolonged study leave scheme have been revised and are available in the current Red Book (SFA 50.1–50.7). Prolonged study leave is not a right, and the quality of your application is important, as it is the only piece of evidence upon which the merits of your application will be judged. Guidelines to the kind of study likely to gain approval are available but are not specific. Your activity or study should be of "value to general practice, or the health service as a whole". A commitment to a written report will gain approval. The most important step is to get good advice and help in preparing your application. Such help should be available from your regional adviser, academic departments of general practice, or other university departments if the study is relevant (for example, medical ethics or the history of medicine). The Scientific Foundation Board of the Royal College of General Practitioners offers expert advice to applicants through their research adviser. Colleagues who have taken extended study leave can also be very useful with advice.

Your application will be submitted to the regional adviser in general practice. It will then go for consideration to the general practitioners' subcommittee and, if approved, then to the postgraduate dean, who will pass it to the Department of Health for consideration and, hopefully, approval. It can take up to 12 weeks for the department to make a decision.

The level of financial support available from the department is subject to guidelines, which can alter from time to time; the postgraduate dean's office will know the current situation. At the time of writing, an allowance for locum expenses is available, but not if the work is covered by the partners without outside help. There is also an educational allowance, which has no strings attached.

Awards, grants and scholarships

Although they are unlikely to cover expenses entailed in taking a sabbatical leave, awards, grants, and scholarships can serve as a very useful passport when visiting other doctors or institutions by lending academic credibility to the visitor. Bodies offering various awards and scholarships include the BMA (Claire Wand Fund), the Royal College of General Practitioners, the World Health Organisation, the King's Fund, the Nuffield Foundation, and the Wellcome Foundation. Some of these awards include travel grants, which are obviously useful if you are considering study abroad.

Exchange of practices

Some doctors have, through personal contacts, exchanged practices with doctors in other countries. Obviously these arrangements remove problems with locum cover. So long as the personalities concerned are compatible, this can be a very good way of gaining a different perspective on medical practice. The difficulty seems to be that integrating the different needs of two doctors and their families can be very complicated. It also has to be said that regulations governing the right to medical practice in different countries, and even different parts of the same country, seem to be getting more complex and more restrictive. Anyone considering an exchange with another doctor needs to check the relevant regulations carefully.

Locums abroad

The range of locum work that may be available to a British doctor seeking sabbatical experience is less extensive than it was, but employment is still available as follows:

General practice locums

There are agencies that arrange for the employment of British doctors in some countries—for instance, Canada, Australia, and

New Zealand. Such agencies will undertake to employ doctors for a definite period. There may be some registration problems in parts of Canada, but this does not yet seem to be a problem for work "down under". Being a locum is not likely to be a relaxed holiday. My partner once did a locum sabbatical near Brisbane, and saw 60 patients a day. One cannot help feeling that the easier locum jobs get filled locally, and agencies advertising abroad are often trying to fill unpopular slots.

International companies

Medical posts with companies or in medical services in the Middle East are advertised regularly in the *BMJ*. Conditions of service should, of course, be scrutinised carefully.

Overseas Development Administration

Medical recruitment by the government's Overseas Development Administration is now much reduced. Work is still available, however, and a local colleague spent three months of 1985 working in the Falklands, where he had lived as a young boy. Such contracts are usually given only for longer periods, but special situations allow for negotiations, and it is always worth a try.

Overseas organisations and agencies

There is still a demand for doctors with specialised skills, and for such people short-term appointments are often possible. For the generalists, suitable work is harder to find, and often requires that the doctor is able to hold an appointment for at least a year. Those interested in exploring the field should first contact the International Health Exchange (see list of addresses and telephone numbers at the end of this chapter), which maintains a register of doctors wishing to work overseas, and publishes a magazine that advertises vacancies. It also organises training courses for those wishing to work abroad and issues a "Short Course Calendar" with details of these courses.

Other agencies listed at the end of this article are also worth contacting, as they often maintain a list of doctors prepared to work for them, and will always give helpful advice.

Of particular interest is a new programme being developed by Voluntary Service Overseas to offer shorter term clinical appointments (3–18 months) in overseas posts, which should suit general practitioners. Doctors interested should contact the organiser of the New Services Unit at Voluntary Service Overseas. The organisation has a selection procedure, and organises funding and appropriate training.

Doing your own thing

Refreshment of spirit seems to me to be the major justification for taking a sabbatical and depriving our patients of our services. We may find ourselves doing the same kind of work as we usually do, though in another setting, but perhaps we should try to do something different—to adopt for a while a new rhythm of life, and perhaps a different identity. I spent a truly recreative year working with the Wellcome Unit of Medical History at Cambridge; others I know have become serious research workers for the first time, medical journalists, or explorers. Some have taken to the arts, music, painting, writing, potting, or other crafts, achieving a new balance in their lives.

Re-entry and splash down

I do not think I should end these thoughts on taking a sabbatical leave without some reflection on the return to work in the practice. To the extent to which the sabbatical has been successful you will have changed. You will not be quite the same doctor, or even perhaps quite the same person, who left the practice. No one should expect to find the re-entry easy. This process is not helped by partners and patients who expect you to be all instant eagerness and fresh energy. As a returning traveller, you will find that everyone else in the practice has fixed their holidays in the confident expectation that you won't really need one. You should not despair. Your sabbatical will, I hope, have stored up treasures for you that will become their own reward once the readjustment is over. Occasionally, of course, the sabbatical is the occasion for a necessary self-examination that provokes a major change in the direction of your professional life. If so, so be it. It is good that such changes should be made while time is still on our side. Otherwise we are in danger of joining what Thoreau thought to be the majority of people, who "lead lives of quiet desperation". So, if you haven't already done so, start planning your sabbatical now—and don't forget to tell your partners and your spouse.

Useful contacts for sabbatical employment abroad

British Red Cross
9 Grosvenor Crescent
London SW1 7EJ
Telephone: 0171-235 5454

Christians Abroad
1 Stockwell Green
London SW9 9HP
Telephone: 0171-737 7811

International Health Exchange
Africa Centre
38 King Street
London WC2E 8JT
Telephone: 0171-836 5833

Overseas Development
  Administration
Abercrombie House
Eaglesham Road
East Kilbride
Glasgow G75 8EA
Telephone: 0171-917 7000 *or*
01355-844000

Oxfam
274 Banbury Road
Oxford OX2 7OZ
Telephone: 01865-311 311
Inquiries to the disaster emergency
officer

Save the Children Fund (Overseas
  Personnel)
Mary Datchelor House
17 Grove Road
Camberwell
London SE5 8RD
Telephone: 0171-703 2278

Voluntary Service Overseas (VSO)
317 Putney Bridge Road
London SW15 2PN
Telephone: 0181-780 2266

III COUNSELLING

32 Broaden your mind about death and related subjects in certain religious groups

John Black

Since the 1950s British society has become diverse in its cultures and religions. Immigration, mainly from the Caribbean, the Indian subcontinent, and East Africa, made a large contribution to these changes. More recently, refugees from political persecution, war, and economic disaster have arrived from Africa, South and Central America, Asia, Eastern Europe and the Middle East. It is possible, though undesirable, to manage an ill person without regard to the patient's ethnic origin, but to be ignorant of the religious beliefs and practices of a dying patient is unforgivable. Much distress and offence can be caused by insensitivity and lack of understanding.

In spite of the changes in the composition of the British population the NHS has paid little attention to the needs of people with faiths other than Christianity, though there have been exceptions, usually at local level. This chapter is an attempt to provide guidance to health workers concerned with the care of dying patients, and to give some information about attitudes to related subjects, such as necropsies, organ transplantation, prenatal testing, termination of pregnancy, and stillbirths.

Administration

Hospitals, clinics and practices in an area with a sizeable population of a particular ethnic or religious group should make appropriate provision for them.[1-3] Areas with inadequate provision, due to small numbers, should seek advice from appropriate centres.

Lists of religious or community leaders, religious centres, appro-

209

priate undertakers, and burial societies, should be available in wards, outpatient and accident and emergency departments, surgeries, and clinics; they should be kept up to date. Explanatory literature about registration of death, burial, necropsies, and stillbirths, and procedures such as prenatal testing, termination of pregnancy, and organ transplantation should be printed in the languages appropriate to the ethnic and religious groups in the area. In areas where the numbers merit it, hospitals should consider the appointment of one or more religious leaders in posts equivalent to that of hospital chaplain.

Symbols of Christianity should be removed from hospital chapels and crematoria when they are used by non-Christians, and sheets used to wrap the body should be plain. Jewellery and other items of possible religious significance should not be removed from the body without the permission of the relatives. In some cultures grief is shown more openly than is the custom in the West, and the provision of a side ward for the dying patient is a humane and sensible gesture. Liaison workers in the hospital or community services can be of great help in these situations.

Buddhism

Buddhism is based on the teachings of Siddhartha Gautama, the Buddha, who lived in the sixth to fifth centuries BC, probably in what is now Nepal. Buddhists believe in rebirth; each individual has led many previous lives, and there is a life after death. People's actions in their life influence the next stage of the rebirth sequence, the aim being to achieve nirvana, perfection. Buddhists are opposed to the taking of all life, not just human life.

Religious organisations

There is no hierarchy in Buddhism except that in monasteries there is a chief monk or abbot. There are no ministers of religion, but monks or sisters are available to give help or advice. There are a number of schools of Buddhism; if possible, inquiries should be made to discover which form of Buddhism a patient belongs to.

Imminent death

The last moments before death are very important. Buddhists should be allowed time for undisturbed meditation, and may refuse pain-relieving drugs in order to keep their mind clear. There are no special rites for the dying, but dying people may be visited by a "spiritual friend" belonging, preferably, to their own school of Buddhism. Buddhists prefer to die at home: a hospital is not a peaceful place.

After death

The body should be wrapped in a plain sheet and should remain undisturbed for the maximum amount of time, to allow the spirit to leave the body; this may be up to three days in Tibetan Buddhism.

Funeral arrangements

Most Buddhists will have informed their relatives of their wishes about funeral arrangements. The body is usually cremated, the ceremony being conducted by the family or a member of the same school of Buddhism.

Mourning

There are no formal rites. The family will do what seems appropriate to them and in accord with the wishes of their dead relative.

Necropsies

Most Buddhists do not approve of necropsy since it involves disturbance of the body. Coroners' necropsies are permitted.

Organ donation and transplant operations

Attitudes to organ donation and transplantation vary; many Buddhists would regard the giving or receiving of an organ as a major disturbance of the body and therefore unacceptable. In Tibetan Buddhism organ donation or transplantation would certainly not be permitted. However, these procedures may be regarded as a method of saving life.

Termination of pregnancy

Because it involves taking life, a Buddhist would not accept termination of a pregnancy.

Prenatal testing

There are no objections to prenatal testing, but this should not be done if there is a possibility of refusal of a termination.

Stillbirths and the death of very young children

Stillborn babies and very young children are treated in the same way as any other person and would therefore be cremated.

Hinduism

The majority of the Hindus in Britain come from Gujarat, in Western India, or from Eastern Africa. Hinduism is a polytheistic religion, embracing a way of life and a social system. Hindus believe in a supreme being residing in each individual, and the ultimate goal is the release of the individual's soul from the cycle of birth, death, and rebirth to join the supreme being. People's deeds in their past lives determine their status and good or ill fortune in their present life, whose quality, in turn, governs their future.

Religious organisation

In Hinduism there is no supreme church authority and no hierarchy. Numerous gods are worshipped, each being the personification of a particular aspect of the supreme being. Most families worship at a shrine in their home, and attend the temple *(mandir)* for communal worship. The temple is in the care of a priest *(pandit, a teacher)*, generally a Brahmin (a member of the highest caste), chosen and supported by the community. The priest has no parochial functions, but may come to the hospital to pray with the relatives of a dying person.

Imminent death

When death is thought to be near, the dying person is given water from the River Ganges (Ganga) and the family or priest read from one of the holy books of Hinduism. The priest may tie a thread round the neck or wrist; this should not be removed. Many Hindu patients prefer to die at home, and this should be respected whenever possible.

After death

Gloves may be required to be worn by non-Hindus when touching or moving the body. The body is generally covered with a plain white sheet, though married Hindu women are often shrouded in red fabric. Usually, the family wishes to wash and lay out the body; this may be done at home, or at an undertaker's.

212

Funeral arrangements

The eldest son is generally responsible for making the funeral arrangements. All Hindus, except stillborn babies and young children (see below) are cremated. In India this is done on the day of death, but the formalities required in Britain make this impracticable; nevertheless, death and cremation certificates should be provided with the least possible delay. Crematorium authorities should ensure the removal of Christian symbols for the service. A well-informed undertaker may be of assistance with the arrangements for the cremation. Ideally, the ashes should be scattered over the waters of the Ganges; but in Britain the ashes are scattered at sea or over any large expanse of water; permission must be obtained for this.

Mourning

The family is in mourning until the thirteenth day after the cremation, when a special ceremony takes place.

Necropsies

Necropsies are not generally approved of, but if legally required by a coroner they are accepted, provided that the situation is fully explained.

Organ donation and transplant operations

There are no religious prohibitions against the giving or receiving of organs.

Termination of pregnancy

The only widely accepted reason for a termination is when an unmarried woman becomes pregnant, although there is considerable variation in attitudes.

Prenatal testing

Since the outcome of a prenatal test may be the advice to terminate the pregnancy, such investigations, whether invasive or not, should not be embarked on without a very full explanation to both parents. It should not, however, be assumed that termination will be refused. The concept of genetic counselling is not widely understood.

Stillbirths and the death of young children

A stillbirth is regarded, from the spiritual point of view, as no different from a child who has lived and then died. Stillborn babies and children under the age of four years (the actual age varies with local custom) are not cremated, as it is held that they cannot stand the heat of cremation and have no awareness of their past actions. Burial can be arranged in a special area of a local cemetery. The formalities for the death of a child vary, but the mourning period and ceremony are usually observed as for an adult.

Islam

"Islam" means submission (to the will of God). A Muslim is a follower of Islam. Most Asian Muslims in Britain have come from Pakistan, Bangladesh, or the Mirpur district of Kashmir (Azad Kashmir); there are also Yamanis, Somalis, and Arabs, and in some cities there are also quite large Turkish and Turkish Cypriot Muslim communities. The Islamic religion was preached by Mohammed, who was born in AD 570 in Mecca (Makka), now in Saudi Arabia. Muslims believe in God (Allah), and that Mohammed is his prophet and messenger. Mohammed is regarded as the last of a long line of prophets, including Abraham, Moses, David, Job, John the Baptist, and Jesus. The Quran consists of the teaching of Islam as revealed to Mohammed, and it together with his recorded sayings and acts constitutes the main sources of the Islamic legal system (Sharia), there being no distinction between religious and secular law. Muslims believe in life after death and that on the day of resurrection people will be judged by God according to their deeds; they will then face everlasting happiness, paradise, or everlasting punishment, hell.

Religious organisation

The mosque (*masjid*) is the centre for worship and religious instruction; it is in the charge of a prayer leader (Imam), who is appointed and supported by the congregation. The Imam is not required to attend the death of a Muslim or to officiate at a burial, because it is everyone's duty to do this, but is usually invited to do so. One should find out whether a patient belongs to the Sunni or Shi'ite branch of Islam.

Imminent death

The family prays at the bedside of the dying person, whose head must be turned towards Mecca; this may entail altering the position of the bed. Dying people are requested to say the Testimony of Islam if it is possible for them to do so.

After death

It is helpful if the orientation of the hospital chapel can be indicated so that the body can be placed with the head towards Mecca. Normally, the body is washed and laid out, either in the mortuary or at the undertaker's, by family members of the same sex as the deceased.

Funeral arrangements

Muslims are buried, and never cremated. Burial should take place as soon after death as possible. The body is taken to the mosque or to the graveside, for prayers. Women may not go to the burial ceremony. Most local authorities provide special areas for Muslim burials. The body is placed in the grave on its right side, facing Mecca. For social and emotional reasons some families take their dead back to their country of origin; this entails much bureaucratic delay, which is very distressing to the relatives, but it is nevertheless the Islamic ideal to be buried in one's place of birth.

Mourning

The bereaved mourn the dead for three days after the funeral. The mourning period prescribed for a widow is four lunar months and ten days; should she be pregnant, the period of mourning ceases when she is delivered.

Necropsies

As the body must not be cut or defaced, routine necropsies are never accepted. Coroners' necropsies are reluctantly accepted if the circumstances are explained to the relatives, and safeguards are given that the organs will not be removed.

Organ donation and transplant operations

Organ donation and transplantation are rarely permitted, but there is much variation in practice. Refusal should not be assumed.

215

According to Shi'ite practice, it is permitted to make a will saying that certain organs may go to a Muslim in need.

Termination of pregnancy

Termination is allowed only in order to save the life of the mother; permission for this should be sought sensitively from the family. In exceptional circumstances, where prenatal testing (especially by non-invasive methods such as ultrasound) has clearly shown that the infant would be born severely handicapped, or suffering from a severe and untreatable disease, the parents may agree to a termination, but only after a committee of consultants has agreed on the diagnosis. However, according to strict Islamic teaching, the taking of life is not permitted even on account of severe fetal disease.

Prenatal testing

Genetic advice is particularly important in Muslim families because of the high proportion of first or second cousin marriages. In a five-year prospective study Bundey and Alam found a three-fold increase in post-neonatal mortality and morbidity in children of consanguineous Pakistani marriages compared to non-consanguineous marriages.[4]

Stillbirths and the death of young children

In general, the body is given to the parents to make the necessary arrangements with the undertaker. It should be noted that after delivery the mother is relieved of all religious acts of worship as long as bleeding continues.

Judaism

In spite of the presence of Jewish communities in Britain since the seventeenth century, there is much ignorance about their beliefs and customs. As with the other major religions, there are numerous subdivisions and sects within Judaism. In general, the differences relate mainly to the degree of observance of traditional practices and rituals. It is important to discover at the earliest opportunity the group to which a patient belongs, since if a rabbi is to be involved he or she (in Reform Judaism the rabbi may be a woman) should belong to the appropriate sect.

There is a spectrum of observance of Jewish teaching and custom, ranging from the minority group of the strictly orthodox Hassidim, to various liberal, reform and progressive groups, in which observance is much less strict. There will also be various degrees of non-observance.

The men of the Hassidic sect are recognisable by their long black coat and trousers and round hat, their beard and long side curls. The women may have their hair cut short and wear a wig, and they usually wear a scarf over their heads. There is a large, closely knit community of Hassidim in north London. Less strictly orthodox men wear a skull cap (*yarmulke*). In general, however, there are no distinguishing marks that characterise a Jew; awareness and sensitive inquiry will establish Jewish adherents and their particular Jewish tradition.

Judaism and Christianity are both monotheistic religions with the same moral base. Both accept that part of the Bible known to Christians as the Old Testament with different emphasis. Judaism does not accept the divinity of Jesus, or the New Testament. Tradition and rituals are based on the Mosaic law (Torah) derived from the Pentateuch (the first five books of the Bible) and the Talmud, which is the fundamental code of Jewish civil and canon law.

For Jews, the Sabbath starts at sunset on Friday and finishes on Saturday evening. No work can be done nor supervised during this period, and deaths occurring on the Sabbath require special arrangements (see below).

Religious organisation

The religious community is centred on the synagogue, and the rabbi, as leader of the congregation. There are Jewish schools, both independent and state subsidised.

Imminent death

A Jew should not die alone. Although there are no last rites in Judaism, when it is evident that death is approaching guardians are present at the bedside to make sure that the dying person receives comfort in the last hours, including the recitation of the confession (*viddui*). The dying may wish to see a rabbi, who will say some prayers with him or her. The relatives derive much support from the presence of a rabbi at this time. It is usually the wish of dying people that someone will say the mourning prayer (*kaddish*) for them.

217

After death

Traditionally, when death is thought to have occurred, the body is left for eight minutes, and a feather is then placed over the mouth and nostrils. If there are no signs of breathing, the eyes and mouth are closed by a son or nearest relative. The arms are extended down the sides of the body, and should not be crossed, and the jaw is bound up. All tubes, instruments, etc, should be removed and incisions plugged. The body is wrapped in a plain cloth and placed on the floor with the feet facing the door and a candle placed at the head. The body should remain there until it is removed for burial. If death occurs on the Sabbath or a festival day, the body should not be moved, but in hospital it should be moved to a room where it remains until taken away for burial. Orthodox procedure watchers (*wachers*) should stay with the body, reciting psalms, until the body is removed for burial. It is recommended that ritual washing of the body (*taharah*) should be performed in addition to the normal washing; this is done by a trained group (*chevra kaddisha*).

Funeral arrangements

According to Jewish practice, the body should be buried as soon as possible; any delay is permissible only for medicolegal reasons. Before burial the body is washed and undergoes a ritual purification practice; this may be omitted in less orthodox communities. The family usually arranges the funeral through a Jewish burial society in the local synagogue.

Burial is obligatory, and cremation is permitted only in some progressive groups or for non-observers. The child of a Jewish mother and a non-Jewish father may be buried in a Jewish cemetery, but not the child of a non-Jewish mother and a Jewish father.

Mourning

Strict mourning (*shivah*) is observed for seven days, during which time the relatives remain at home and receive visitors. Shivah is not observed for infants dying within 30 days of birth. Mourning rituals must be observed by boys of 13 years and one day, and by girls of 12 years and one day.

Necropsies

For orthodox Jews necropsies are accepted only if ordered by the coroner for medicolegal purposes. The organs must be replaced in

218

the body. The prohibition against necropsies can be overridden if the examination would help in the saving of life in the future (for example, for research purposes).

Organ donation and transplant operations

In general, donation and transplantation are permitted if life will be saved by the procedure; this includes the donation from a living person (a kidney) if the donor's life is not endangered. Corneal transplantation is also normally permitted.

Amputation

Amputated limbs are considered as intrinsic parts of the body and should be formally buried.

Termination of pregnancy

For orthodox Jews, termination is generally allowed only if the mother's health or life would be endangered by continuing the pregnancy. Some authorities permit termination for fetal abnormality, which should be performed under 40 days. Jewish practice is, in general, compatible with the abortion legislation in England and Wales.

Prenatal testing

If the parents would not accept a termination if it were to be advised as a result of the test, then prenatal tests should not be performed.

Stillbirths and the death of young children

Judaism does not consider a stillbirth or a child dying under the age of 30 days to have existed and therefore does not require a burial service or a headstone. In the Reform movement it is recognised that a formal recognition of the child's death helps the parents to accept the death and to grieve; in the circumstances a service is permitted and a shortened mourning period.

Sikhism

The Sikhs in Britain have come from the state of Punjab in India, or from Eastern Africa. The word Sikh means disciple or follower. The Sikh religion was founded by a Hindu, Guru Nanak (1469–1539), who reacted against the excessive ritual, the priestly dominance, and the caste system of Hinduism. Sikhs believe in one god, and Guru Nanak is revered as a man chosen by God to reveal his message. In Sikhism men and women are equal.

Religious organisation

There are no ordained priests in Sikhism; the Sikh temple (*gurdwara*) is in the care of a reader (*granthi*), who is appointed and supported by the community. The gurdwara may also be used as a social and advice centre, and for children's classes in religion and Punjabi.

Imminent death

When a person is close to death, the family, sometimes accompanied by the granthi, pray at the bedside and read from the holy book, the Guru Granth Sahib.

After death

The Sikhs have no objection to the body being touched by non-Sikhs. The family usually lay out and wash the body themselves.

Funeral arrangements

The body is taken to the undertaker's by way of the family home, where the coffin is opened so that the dead person may be seen for the last time. All Sikh men and women, in life and after death, must wear the five signs of Sikhism; these are *kesh*, uncut hair (and beard); the *kangha*, a semicircular comb that fixes the uncut hair in a bun; the *kara*, a steel or, occasionally, gold bangle worn on the right wrist; the *kirpan*, a symbolic dagger worn under the clothes in a small cloth sheath or simply a kirpan-shaped brooch or pendant; the *kaccha*, long undershorts reaching to the knees, now often replaced by ordinary underpants, which have the same significance. Sikh men wear their turban after death.

All Sikhs, apart from stillborn babies and infants dying within a few days of birth, are cremated. The ashes are scattered at sea or in a river, or they may be taken to a holy place, commonly the River Sutlej at Anandpur, where Sikhism was founded.

Mourning

The family is in mourning for about 10 days, though this varies. The end of mourning is marked by a ceremony (*Bhaug*) held at the

220

family home. For children under the age of eight or nine years the arrangements tend to be less formal.

Necropsies

There is no religious objection to necropsies, but there may be some resistance to the idea from families originating in rural Punjab, where these would not be usual.

Organ donation and transplant operations

These are accepted.

Termination of pregnancy

This is not generally approved except where an unmarried woman becomes pregnant.

Prenatal testing

Though there are no religious objections to this, the idea of amniocentesis or fetal blood sampling may be unfamiliar and require considerable explanation. In any case, invasive investigations on the fetus should not be done if there is no likelihood of a termination being accepted.

Stillbirths and the death of young children

The bodies of stillborn babies or infants who have died within a few days of birth are usually buried. The arrangements are similar to those for Hindu infants.

Helping or counselling?

Nursing staff in particular can be of great help in advising bereaved and bewildered relatives on the procedures for registration of death, cremation certificates, and finding a suitable undertaker. The hospital chaplain may take on these duties and may be able to put relatives in touch with members of their own religion or community when no relatives are easily accessible. In discussions with some of the (male) leaders of the Hindu, Sikh, and Islamic communities I have not received the impression that there is a need for bereavement counsellors. It is difficult to obtain the women's viewpoint on this, as traditionally, and often for linguistic reasons, the man speaks for his wife. It is, however, often acceptable for another woman to talk to a bereaved mother. The Stillbirth and

Neonatal Death Society has often been of help to bereaved families, in spite of linguistic and cultural differences.

Acknowledgements

I am grateful to the following for their help and advice: Hadji Haslam Ali, The Islamic Mosque, Whitechapel Road, London; Dr S Nutawalli Darsh, London; Pandit Mathoor Krishnamurti, Institute of Indian Culture, London; Dr S Fadil Milani, Al-Khoei Foundation, London; Mr B C Rosenberg, Sheffield; Professor C P Seager, University of Sheffield; Mr Jaspar Singh Bamra, Southall; Dr Suha Taji-Farouki, University of Durham; Mr R Wills, The Buddhist Hospice Trust, London.

1 Black J. NHS hik hai? *BMJ* 1984; **289**: 1558–9.
2 Black J. *Child health in a multicultural society: new paediatrics.* 2nd ed. London: *BMJ*, 1989; 7–17.
3 Winkler F, Yung J. Advising Asian mothers. *Health and Social Services Journal* 1981; **91**: 1244–5.
4 Bundey S, Alam H. A five-year prospective study of the health of children in different ethnic groups, with particular reference to the effect of inbreeding. *Eur J Hum Genet* 1993; **1**: 206–19.

Further reading

Henley A. *Asian patients in hospital and at home.* London: Pitman Medical, 1979.
Henley A. *Asians in Britain: caring for Muslims and their families; religious aspects of care.* Cambridge: National Extension College, 1982.
Henley A. *Asians in Britain: caring for Hindus and their families; religious aspects of care.* Cambridge: National Extension College, 1983.
Henley A. *Asians in Britain: caring for Sikhs and their families; religious aspects of care.* Cambridge: National Extension College, 1983.
Hospital Chaplaincy Council. *Our ministry and other faiths.* London: CIO Publishing, 1983.
Islamic World League. *Funeral arrangements in Islam.* Dar Al-Kitab Al-Masri, 33 Kasr El-Nil Street, Cairo, Egypt (obtainable from some mosques in Britain).
Neuberger J. *Caring for dying people of different faiths.* Lisa Sainsbury Foundation Series, London: Austen Cornish, 1987.
Rabinowicz H. *A guide to life: Jewish laws and customs of mourning.* London: Jewish Chronicle Publications, 1982.
Sampson C. *The neglected ethic: religious and cultural factors in the care of patients.* London: McGraw-Hill, 1982.
Walter C. Attitudes to death and bereavement among cultural minority groups. *Nursing Times* 1982; Dec.15: 2106–9.
Wright M. *A death in the family.* Guernsey: Guernsey Press Company, 1987.

33 Improve the counselling skills of doctors and nurses in cancer care

Peter Maguire, Ann Faulkner

The diagnosis and treatment of cancer cause considerable psychological distress and morbidity.[1] But this is resolved in only a minority of patients because those concerned in their care tend to avoid the emotional aspects.[2] They distance themselves for three main reasons:

(1) They lack the skills to handle the difficult problems and strong emotions that may emerge if they talk with patients and relatives in any depth.

(2) They fear that probing into how a person is adjusting psychologically will cause harm.

(3) They are concerned that there will not be practical or psychological support available to them in this more psychological role.[3]

Fortunately, many doctors and nurses who care for cancer patients realise that their difficulties in communicating with patients and relatives stem from insufficient training and are eager to remedy this. In this chapter we describe how to run short intensive workshops to help doctors and nurses improve their skills in interviewing, assessment, and counselling.

Structure

Participants

Nurses often complain that they cannot talk openly with cancer patients because doctors will not let them do so and that doctors ignore important feedback about patients. Doctors usually counter

223

these complaints by stating that nurses are too eager to "pass the buck" to them and do not understand how difficult it is to break bad news and initiate unpleasant treatments. Doctors and nurses are, therefore, both included in the workshops so that these opposing views can be aired, discussed, and resolved. Attempts are made to ensure equal representation of hospital and community staff, for the latter tend to excuse their reluctance to talk with cancer patients on the basis that they still have to hear formally from the hospital what patients have been told about their illness and prognosis.

Size

The workshops are limited to 16 people so that participants are involved fully and have several opportunities to practise their skills and receive feedback in small groups.

Setting

The workshops are held away from the main hospital so that participants won't be contacted to deal with clinical problems. Rooms are selected that allow both large and small group work to be conducted in comfort. A good standard of catering is also important. This allows participants to devote their attention to the workshops instead of complaining about the setting and food.

Duration

Three days are needed to cover the main agenda and permit discussion about how to apply newly acquired skills while ensuring personal survival.

Teaching

Tutors

The workshops require experienced doctors and nurses to acknowledge that they find certain counselling situations hard to cope with because they lack the relevant skills. They also have to watch demonstration videotapes that show patients and relatives in various predicaments. Strong feelings may be aroused and powerful memories triggered. Only one facilitator leads these demonstration sessions so that the other three facilitators can monitor reactions and intervene publicly or privately when necessary in order to minimise

224

the risk that participants will be harmed. It also allows potentially damaging situations to be used constructively, as in the following example.

While an experienced general practitioner watched a videotape of an interview between a facilitator (PM) and a woman with advanced breast cancer, she became very angry and accused him of "emotional rape". She argued that the considerable distress that the woman disclosed was caused by the facilitator's interviewing style. Her anger seemed out of all proportion to the reality portrayed on the tape. The key facilitator first invited her in the larger session to discuss why she was reacting that way. She declined to do so and therefore, after the session, the facilitator of her small group sought her out for a private conversation. The general practitioner disclosed that her mother had recently been treated for breast cancer and had developed serious emotional problems. She was very angry about this because she believed they were a direct consequence of poor medical management.

Methods

It is crucial that teaching methods are congruent with the models of interviewing, assessment, and counselling being taught. For this reason the beginning of each workshop mirrors the initial phase of an assessment interview with a patient who has requested help. (Key techniques are in parentheses.)

Beginning

The facilitators introduce themselves (self-introduction), give the aims of the workshop, and the methods that will be used (orientation), and check if these are acceptable (negotiation). The facilitators stress that they are willing to adapt the methods to meet the participants' particular needs (sensitivity to individual needs). Participants are then asked to explain who they are, why they have come, and what they are hoping for from the workshops (establishing expectations).

They are next asked to think of and disclose problems they have experienced in recent weeks when talking to cancer patients, relatives, and colleagues that they would like to have handled better. They are split into two small groups of eight to do this. Each group appoints a leader, who ensures that each participant contributes at least one problem (promoting honest disclosure of key problems).

225

Another member keeps a record of the problems (recording key problems). It is emphasised that the success of the workshop depends, like counselling, on the level of their disclosures. If important problems remain hidden, they cannot be discussed and resolved.

When the group reconvenes, a rapporteur from each group describes the problems that have been disclosed. The nature and extent of each problem offered is then clarified by inviting the participant who volunteered the problem to give more detail (clarification, precision). As each problem is clarified it is listed on a flipchart (compiling a problem list). After all the problems have been mentioned the participants are asked if there are any other problems they would like help with (screening for any other problems).

Agreeing the goals

As in real life, there may be too many problems to cover in the time available. Priorities have to be decided and realistic goals set. Participants are asked in turn to rate how essential it is for them to cover each listed problem on a scale from 0 or no relevance to 10 or most essential. They are advised to think only of their own needs and work situation when giving a rating verbally (disclosing real versus expected needs). Group scores are calculated for each problem (range 0 to 160). Problems are then relisted on a flipchart in rank order from the most to least essential.

The agenda of the workshop is decided on the basis of the top eight problems (table I). The problems to be covered are summarised by a facilitator and the group is asked if this agenda is acceptable (summarise goals, check acceptability). It is then explained that the other problems listed will be dealt with in a later session (reviewing unfinished business).

Basic interviewing and assessment

The teaching first focuses on the least difficult problem first in order to generate confidence. This is invariably how to establish quickly an empathic relationship with a patient and identify key problems. A videotape showing a facilitator conducting an assessment is used to show the aspects to be covered and the skills to be used. Facilitators are exposed to such scrutiny to emphasise that they are not perfect interviewers or counsellors and can tolerate and heed constructive feedback.

226

TABLE I Problem list

	Score (maximum = 200)	% of maximum possible
Breaking bad news	180	90.0
Patient who has been lied to	178	89.0
Basic interviewing/assessment	177	88.5
Handling difficult questions	175	87.5
Dealing with the angry patient	171	85.5
Challenging denial	168	84.0
Sudden, unexpected death	163	81.5
Bereaved relatives	158	79.0
Breaking collusion	153	76.5
Handling the withdrawn patient	149	74.5

The aspects covered are history of the patient's illness and treatment to date; patient's perceptions, psychological reactions and view of the future; and impact of illness and treatment on the patient's daily life, mood, and key relationships. Techniques that have been found to promote disclosure are emphasised: asking open directive questions ("How have you felt about losing a breast?"), acknowledging, organising, clarifying and exploring key verbal and non-verbal cues; how to keep patients to the point and use time optimally but avoid alienation; encouraging precise accounts of their experiences so that patients make the effort to remember and describe these and the associated feelings fully and accurately; encouraging the expression of feelings through the use of empathy and educated guesses about how the patient is feeling; summarising what has been heard so far and screening for any other problems.

Key strategies shown are how to deal with patients' concerns before professional concerns—like review of physical systems; ensuring full coverage of one topic before moving to another—for example, the nature and extent of a body image problem before talking about the partner's responses; obtaining a list of all key problems before giving advice or attempting any resolution; and how to help the patient move in and out of strong emotions. The tapes are stopped at key points and participants invited to suggest which topics are being covered and why, which techniques and strategies are being used, and the emotional level of the interview (0 = neutral, 1 = hint of feeling, 2 = explicit mention of feeling, 3 = expression of feelings). The interviewing and assessment model is thus made explicit and the participants build up a vocabulary that will allow them to analyse their interviews during the rest of the workshop.

After participants have assimilated the model, they are split into four groups, each with a facilitator, to practise basic interviewing and assessment skills by role play.

Use of role play

Role play allows participants to practise under controlled conditions, and audiotape recording permits playback and discussions. Otherwise much time can be lost in debating whether or not certain skills were used. Most participants are wary of role play because of adverse experiences. They are asked to disclose these and consider why the experience was unpleasant. The ground rules for the methods of role play to be used in the workshop are then explained. These include observing the following rules:

(1) Every participant will do a role play.

(2) The patient, relative, or colleague presenting the problem will be played by the person who volunteered it as a difficult problem in the initial small group discussions.

(3) A participant should not play a particular role—for example, a bereaved relative—if it is too close to an adverse personal experience (bereavement).

(4) The role player will not make the problem more difficult than it was in real life.

(5) The doctor or nurse tackling the problem will be given an explicit, simple but realistic brief.

(6) Each role player will stay within the brief given.

(7) If the participant feels stuck in the role play he or she must call time out, otherwise the facilitator will do so to avoid embarrassment and humiliation.

(8) When a role play is stopped, the doctor or nurse and the person playing a patient, relative, or colleague will first be asked to comment on how he or she thinks the interaction is going.

(9) Other members of the group will then be asked to identify strengths in the performance of the doctor or nurse.

(10) Only when they have exhausted all strengths, will they be allowed by the facilitator to suggest why the doctor or nurse got stuck.

(11) The group (not the doctor or nurse) will be asked to offer other strategies.

(12) The doctor or nurse will then be invited to test out these strategies in role play until the problem is resolved.

228

Briefing

The participant playing the patient, relative, or colleague is taken out of the room and briefed by a facilitator, who uses the participant's real-life experience of the problem to develop the brief. The role player then returns to the room to sit down and "get into role" while the facilitator briefs the doctor or nurse. For example: Sheila is a 32-year-old housewife who was told two years ago that her breast cancer had been cured by surgery and radiotherapy. She has now developed a recurrence on her scar line and has widespread bony metastases. She has been referred to you as a medical oncologist for advice about further treatment. Your task is to assess her and determine her current problems and whether they are physical, social or psychological. Remember to signal time out if you feel stuck and the facilitator will then ask the group to suggest alternative strategies.

Feedback

The doctor then joins the "patient" and is asked to begin the role play by asking an open question—for example, what problems have brought you here today? The facilitator starts the audiotape recording and the role play continues until time out is signalled by the doctor or facilitator, usually some three or four minutes later. Each participant in the role play is asked to comment on how it is going, emphasising good points first. The group is then requested to highlight what they liked. Only when no more strengths are forthcoming are constructive criticisms invited by the facilitator, who asks: "Why did the doctor get stuck?" The facilitator asks the group to suggest what other strategies might be tried (emphasising a shared approach to problem solving). These strategies are then discussed and tested out in further role play (testing out strategies). The facilitator resists offering a solution unless the group fails to resolve the problem (encouraging participants to generate their own solutions). These exercises in role play concerning basic interviewing and assessments are carried out in sessions lasting 75 to 90 minutes (table II).

Problems in counselling

Role play is also used to help participants to learn how to resolve other problems on the main agenda, such as breaking bad news and relating to an angry patient. Explicit briefs are given based on real-

TABLE II Timetable and agenda for workshop

Day 1

8.45 am	Registration and coffee
9.00 am	Introduction
9.30 am	Base line skills: Group A
	Agenda setting: Group B
10.30 am	Coffee
11.00 am	Agenda setting: Group A
	Base line skills: Group B
12.00 pm	Agreeing the agenda
1.00 pm	Lunch
2.00 pm	Key assessment skills (demonstration and discussion)
3.30 pm	Tea
4.00 pm	Key assessment skills continued
5.30 pm	Close

Day 2

9.00 am	Unfinished business from day 1
9.30 am	Dealing with difficult situations
	Small group work (role play)
10.45 am	Coffee
11.15 am	Small group work (role play)
12.45 pm	Lunch
2.00 pm	Small group work (role play)
3.30 pm	Tea
4.00 pm	Videotape demonstrations
5.30 pm	Close

Day 3

9.00 am	Unfinished business from day 2
9.30 am	Dealing with difficult situations
	Small group work (role play)
10.45 am	Coffee
11.15 am	Unfinished business
12.00 pm	Survival issues
1.00 pm	Lunch
2.00 pm	Evaluation: Group A
	Post course skills: Group B
3.00 pm	Post course skills: Group A
	Evaluation: Group B
4.00 pm	Tea
4.30 pm	Close

life situations disclosed by the participants. For example: John has a lymphoma diagnosed two years ago and was treated with chemotherapy and radiotherapy. He experienced severe adverse effects, particularly conditioned vomiting. He nearly opted out but was persuaded to continue by the argument that he had a 95% chance of a complete cure. His lymphoma has returned and further chemotherapy has been suggested. He feels very angry and is refusing treatment.

John is played by the doctor who encountered this predicament. This gives the doctor valuable insight into what it might have been like to be on the receiving end of care.

These problems are covered in subsequent sessions (table II), which, like counselling, can be intense and emotionally draining but enriching. They are separated by coffee and lunch breaks (need for time out) and further videotape demonstrations that are both serious and humorous (need for light relief). The role playing is distributed equitably within each group so that no one takes an undue burden (sharing the load).

Ending

Unfinished business

After completion of the agreed goals the unfinished business is reviewed.

Survival

Participants are invited to discuss the fears and concerns they have about trying to apply their new skills when they return to their place of work. Particular emphasis is placed on their own attitudes to death and dying, personal involvement with the patient and how to handle strong emotions, and the importance of sharing concerns promptly with colleagues whether formally in support groups or informally.

Review

Participants are asked to say what they found most and least helpful in the workshop (asking for feedback), and to suggest improvements (demonstrate willingness to learn).

Follow up

A one and a half day workshop is usually held six months later to discuss how far participants have been able to apply what they learned and obtain adequate support. It also allows them to discuss if their new skills were effective (validation) and to practise more difficult counselling tasks.

Discussion

These workshops, which are supported by the Cancer Research Campaign, are attempting to meet an important need for training in counselling skills. An analysis of audiotapes of the role playing in the workshops has confirmed that this need is real and substantial. All the facilitators continue to be impressed by the willingness of experienced doctors and nurses to subject themselves to such close scrutiny, for it is hard for such experienced professionals to admit to being inadequate in respect of their interviewing and assessment skills. Fortunately, the feedback from participants has been consistently positive and most have claimed they have improved their skills and become more confident. This has been confirmed by recent research that has examined the extent to which the interviewing skills of participants have changed in the short and longer term.

1 Greer S. Cancer: psychiatric aspects. In Granville-Grossman K, ed. *Recent advances in clinical psychiatry*. London: Churchill Livingstone, 1985; 87–103.
2 Maguire P. Barriers to psychological care of the dying. *BMJ* 1985; **291**: 1711–13.
3 Wilkinson S. Factors which influence how nurses communicate with cancer patients. *J of Advanced Nursing* 1991; **16**: 677–88.

34 Communicate with cancer patients: 1 Handling bad news and difficult questions

Peter Maguire, Ann Faulkner

In this chapter we suggest how to handle situations in communicating with patients with cancer that doctors and nurses commonly find difficult.[1]

Breaking bad news

It is important to accept that you cannot soften the impact of bad news, since it is still bad news however it is broken. The first step is to check the level of the patient's awareness of the reality of his or her condition. This can be done by asking, for example, "Have you had any thoughts about what these symptoms might be due to?" The majority of patients have a good awareness that they have cancer and so will respond to questions by signalling that they realise that it could be serious. The breaking of bad news is then a matter of confirming their awareness rather than giving them unexpected news.

An important minority of patients have no idea of the potential seriousness of their condition. The key to breaking bad news to them is to try to slow down the speed of transition from their perception of themselves as being well to a realisation that they have a life-threatening disease. If you break the news too abruptly, it will disorganise them psychologically and they will have difficulty adapting. They may become overwhelmed with distress. Alternatively, it may provoke denial because the news is too painful to assimilate. Thus you should avoid stating boldy, "I am afraid you have got cancer" and instead warn that you are about to communicate some serious information by saying, for example, "I am afraid it looks more serious than an ulcer".

While you may be tempted immediately to soften this bad news by adding, "Even so we should still be able to do something about it", resist this and pause to let your warning sink in. This will also allow you time to monitor how your patient is reacting. What you say next depends on the patient's response. A question like "What do you mean, not just an ulcer?" suggests that the person wants more information. However, a patient who says, "That's all right, doctor, I'll leave it up to you," is suggesting that he or she does not wish to learn any more at this time. By using a hierarchy of euphemisms for the word cancer, such as "a few odd cells", "a kind of tumour", "a bit cancerous", it is possible to manage the transition so that you can establish at each step whether your patient wants to go further in the truth-telling process or not.

Doctor:	I'm afraid it's more than just an ulcer . . .
Mr K:	What do you mean, more than just an ulcer?
Doctor:	Some of the cells looked abnormal under the microscope.
Mr K:	Abnormal?
Doctor:	They looked cancerous.
Mr K:	You mean I've got cancer?
Doctor:	I am afraid so, yes.

When you have either confirmed that the patient's awareness that his or her condition is serious is correct or have broken the bad news, it is important to acknowledge and explore the basis for his or her responses. This will usually reveal that there are good reasons for them.

Doctor:	I can see this news has upset you. Can you bear to say just how you are feeling?
Mr K:	Terrified! I've always had this thing about cancer. I have always been frightened of getting it. Two of my uncles died of it. They both had a bad time. Suffered terrible pain and wasted away . . . to nothing.
Doctor:	So, you're frightened you're going to go the same way.

Mr K:	I'm bound to be scared, aren't I?
Doctor:	Yes, you are, in view of those experiences. It must be hard for you. Any other reasons why you are terrified?
Mr K:	I hate being a burden. My wife has enough to contend with as it is.

Having established the patient's immediate responses, you should establish any other concerns before attempting to give any information about the treatment you propose and the likely outcome. Otherwise these concerns will not be disclosed, the individual will remain preoccupied with them, and in consequence will not heed your advice, and may misperceive what you say. Moreover, it has been found that the number of undisclosed and unresolved concerns is a powerful predictor of subsequent psychiatric morbidity, including adjustment disorders, generalised anxiety disorder, and major depressive illness. It is important that you remember at this stage that what patients want is to feel that their concerns have been understood and may be resolved in the foreseeable future, rather than immediately.

Doctor:	We have explored why you feel so terrified knowing you have cancer. Has it caused you to have any other worries?
Mr C:	Yes.
Doctor:	Would you like to tell me about them?
Mr C:	I am not sure whether I should go ahead with my plans to move house.
Doctor:	It sounds as though you are worried that we may not be able to do anything for your cancer.
Mr C:	Yes, I am.
Doctor:	I'll come back to that in a minute. Before I do, do you have any other concerns?
Mr C:	Yes. Who will look after the children if I don't make it?
Doctor:	So, you are worried about whether or not to move house, and about your children.
Mr C:	Yes, I am.
Doctor:	Anything else you're concerned about?
Mr C:	No.
Doctor:	Are you sure?

Mr C:	Yes, isn't that enough?
Doctor:	It is important I check that I have given you a chance to tell me all your current worries.

When you have established your patient's concerns, you should help the patient put these in priority order, particularly if time is short.

Doctor:	So, you feel you have been able to tell me all your current concerns?
Mrs H:	Yes.
Doctor:	Could you say which of your concerns is bothering you most?
Mrs H:	It's the prospect of pain that terrifies me.
Doctor:	Can you say why that is?
Mrs H:	My mother had the same cancer and died in terrible pain, so I am terrified the same thing will happen to me.
Doctor:	Just how terrifying is this?
Mrs H:	It's uppermost in my mind at the moment.
Doctor:	So, shall we talk about this issue of pain first?
Mrs H:	Yes.

It is important that doctors make sure that their statements about such a concern are realistic but maintain hope. Thus they might say "There is every chance that we can do something for your pain. It is very important you let me know if you develop any pain, then we can see what we can do. Is that all right?"

Often the patient's main concern at the point of breaking bad news or having awareness confirmed is to hear about the extent of the cancer and whether treatment is likely to work. Here again it is important to make statements that are realistic but foster and maintain hope.

Doctor:	When we removed your cancer we found that a few of the nodes under your arm were affected and we removed those as well. To be sure we mop up all the cancer we ought to give you some chemotherapy. There is then a good chance you will be OK.
Mrs M:	You are not certain?

Doctor: No, I can't be certain, but I do think there is every chance of a reasonable outcome in your case providing you have some chemotherapy.

When the prognosis is poor the doctor can usually indicate that something can be done.

Doctor: You are right, you have got lung cancer.

Mr S: That's what I thought, I keep coughing up blood and I have lost so much weight. Are you going to be able to do anything about it?

Doctor: Yes, I think so. I am hopeful that we will get some response from radiotherapy and you will feel much less ill.

Mr S: Only some response?

Doctor: Well, we should be able to shrink it considerably, I am not certain we would be able to get it all.

Mr S: You mean some could be left?

Doctor: There could be. But we would then consider giving you a course of strong drugs. I think we ought to start with radiotherapy first. I am pretty certain we can get it under control and that will make you feel better.

Mr S: I suppose I have to be grateful for that.

Doctor: I can understand that you are disappointed that I can't guarantee getting rid of it all but I think it likely you will feel better once you start radiotherapy. Then maybe you won't be so worried. We still have the drugs at our disposal should they be necessary.

Even when you cannot eradicate the disease it is still important to explore your patients' concerns and associated feelings since it is important that they feel that these are understood and it is likely that you can still do something positive about some of them.

GP: You remember that you came to see me because you were feeling so weak and were worried your cancer had come back and was spreading . . . and I sent you to the hospital for tests?

Mr F: Yes, I do.

237

GP: Good. The reason I came round this morning was to give you the results of those tests they did at the hospital.

Mr F: Yes, I guessed that. What did they find?

GP: I am afraid your guess was right, the cancer has come back. That's the reason why you have been feeling so weak and tired.

Mr F: I thought so. Are you going to be able to do anything for me?

GP: I'm afraid I do not feel that further treatment is going to make much difference to the cancer.

The general practitioner then explored Mr F's resulting concerns and an important issue emerged. He was worried that he might suffer severe pain.

GP: I am sorry to have to tell you this. It can't be easy for you. Do you have any particular worries?

Mr F: I am terrified of getting bad pain.

GP: Just how terrified are you?

Mr F: I can't sleep at night for thinking about it. It's dominating my thinking. It is making me extremely anxious and tense.

GP: Just how tense?

Mr F: I can't relax. I have also got very irritable.

GP: Well, clearly I need to try to help you with this anxiety. If you do get any pain, I hope we will be able to control it with strong painkillers. Let me know the moment you have any problems with pain, or any other symptoms, come to that. The sooner we know about any problems, the sooner we should be able to try to do something.

Mr F: Yes, I can see that.

GP: Apart from getting pain, are there any other concerns?

Mr F: No.

GP: I am sorry it has worked out this way, but we certainly should be able to do something to help you if there are any problems with pain. It is very important we keep in close touch.

The doctor did not say the pain could be eliminated, for this would be false reassurance. Instead, the doctor indicated that there was every chance the pain could be palliated, and showed that he was prepared to discuss other concerns.

This strategy of acknowledging and exploring the emotional response to the bad news and the concerns that contribute to that distress is vital if the breaking of bad news is to be managed effectively. It allows the patient to be "lifted" from being overwhelmed by the news to feeling distressed but hopeful that something can be done.

The key is to maintain a momentum so that patients don't sink so deeply into distress that they can't be rescued. This is achieved by acknowledging the distress and asking patients to explain why they are feeling so distressed and to identify the component concerns and feelings. Patients may change the topic first to avoid undue distress. Alternatively, interviewers may do so when they feel they have understood the nature and extent of a specific concern and the associated feelings. Doctors who are unsure about this should consult the patient.

Doctor:	We have discussed how devastated you feel at knowing you have got a cancer that is incurable, particularly as you have got a young family. Do you feel I have understood sufficiently how you feel about that?
Mrs D:	Yes, I do.
Doctor:	Is it all right then if I move on to check if you have any other concerns?
Mrs D:	Yes, that's all right.

Handling difficult questions

Many doctors and nurses fear that if they get into a dialogue with patients with cancer they will be asked difficult questions—for example, "Is it cancer?"[2] When such a question is asked, it is difficult to know what response is wanted by patients. Do they want the reassurance that it isn't cancer (because they want to deny the reality of the illness) or do they want the truth? Only the patients can suggest the direction they wish to follow. You can usually discover this by saying, "I would be happy to answer your question" and then reflecting the question back to the patient by asking "But what makes you ask that question?" You should then explore if there are other reasons why the person asked it. It will then become clear the patient is asking the question because he or she has guessed what is going on and wants confirmation.

Mr M:	Is it cancer?
Specialist nurse:	I would be happy to answer your questions, but can I first ask why you're asking me?
Mr M:	It's obvious, isn't it?
Specialist nurse:	Why obvious?
Mr M:	I have lost two stone in weight. I'm feeling weaker day by day, and still coughing up blood. It's got to be cancer.
Specialist nurse:	Any other reasons why you are so sure that you've got cancer?
Mr M:	I've been a heavy smoker all of my life. The doctors want to give me radiotherapy. You only get radiotherapy for one thing and that's cancer.
Specialist nurse:	Yes, I'm afraid you're right.
Mr M:	I knew it, I'm not a fool. Why did they tell me they were just giving me radiotherapy as an insurance?
Specialist nurse:	I honestly don't know. But look, would you like to talk more about it?
Mr M:	Yes, I would. What I really want to know—is radiotherapy going to make any difference?
Specialist nurse:	We're hopeful that it will get the cancer under control and that some of the symptoms you're complaining about will improve considerably.
Mr M:	That sounds better than I thought. I thought I was a goner.
Specialist nurse:	A goner?
Mr M:	I thought I'd only a few days to live at most.
Specialist nurse:	That's not the case. There is a real prospect that the treatment will help you feel better and keep you going for some time.

Some patients indicate that they wish to deny what is happening.

Mrs R:	I'm going to get better, aren't I?
Oncologist:	What makes you ask that?
Mrs R:	You and your team tell me that I have some kind of lymphoma. I can't accept that. I'm certain it is an infection I picked up when I was out in the tropics.

Oncologist:	I don't want to argue with you about that. The key thing is that you continue with our treatment.
Mrs R:	I'm happy to do that.

Conclusion

You may have noticed that the strategies we advise are determined by the patient's responses and not decided unilaterally by the doctor or nurse. We do not expect you to accept them unquestioningly, but hope you will try them out with patients in your care. You should then learn that they allow bad news to be broken effectively and difficult questions to be answered without provoking denial or disorganising the patient.

Acknowledgement

This chapter is based on work funded by the Cancer Research Campaign.

1 Maguire P, Faulkner A. How to do it: Improve the counselling skills of doctors and nurses in cancer care. *BMJ* 1988; **297**: 847–9.
2 Maguire P. Barriers to psychological care of the dying. *BMJ* 1985; **291**: 1711–13.

35 Communicate with cancer patients: 2 Handling uncertainty, collusion, and denial

Peter Maguire, Ann Faulkner

Breaking bad news often prompts patients to ask questions about their future, like "How long have I got?" You then have to help them cope with the inevitable uncertainty without them becoming demoralised.

Handling uncertainty

When asked "How long have I got?" it is tempting to give a finite answer ("Oh, three months") or range of time ("Anything from a month to six months"). But such predictions are usually inaccurate, tend to err on the optimistic side, and cause problems for patients and their families. Patients then pace themselves according to the time they believe is left. If they deteriorate earlier than expected and are prevented from achieving planned goals, they will feel cheated and bitter. Relatives can find an unexpectedly prolonged survival ("borrowed time") hard to cope with because they have used up their physical and emotional resources. So it is better to acknowledge your uncertainty and the difficulties that this will cause.

Doctor:	You asked me how long he has. The trouble is, I don't know. I realise this uncertainty must be difficult for you.
Mrs W:	It is. It is terrible knowing that he is going to die but not knowing when. I mean it could be in one month's time or next Christmas.
Doctor:	That's the trouble, I just don't know how long it will be.

You should next check if she would like to know the signs and symptoms that would herald further deterioration.

Doctor: What I can do, but only if you would like me to, is tell you what changes would suggest he is beginning to deteriorate further.

Mrs W: Yes, I think that would help me.

Doctor: He will probably complain of feeling breathless and weak, and start going off his food.

You can then encourage her to try to use the intervening time.

Doctor: But as long as there are no signs like that I think you can take it that he is relatively OK. So, you should try to make the most of this time if you can. Is there anything you would particularly like to do?

Later, add that you are prepared to check him regularly, and show a willingness to negotiate the frequency of such check ups.

Doctor: I think it would help if I saw him from time to time to monitor how he is doing. How often would you like me to do that?

Mrs W: Would every month be OK?

Doctor: Yes, fine.

You should explain that if anything unforeseen occurs between these assessments you should be contacted immediately. This gives patients and relatives confidence that they have a "lifeline".

Doctor: If you are worried at any stage between his appointments you must get in touch with me. I can then assess him and decide what needs to be done.

Few patients or relatives abuse this offer.

When some patients or relatives face uncertainty, they show that they do not want any markers.

Doctor: Would you like me to tell you how you might recognise if Peter's health is deteriorating?

Mrs B: No, I'll leave it to you. You're the expert.

Sometimes the uncertainty concerns issues other than "how long". Again, you should acknowledge the uncertainty and establish any resulting worries.

Doctor:	I sense that this uncertainty is a major problem for you.
Mr J:	It is. I feel helpless not knowing what's going to happen or how it's going to happen.
Doctor:	What are you worried about in particular?
Mr J:	I'm worried about how I'm going to die. I don't want to be a burden on my family, and I'm not sure what to expect after death.
Doctor:	Any other concerns?
Mr J:	Isn't that enough?
Doctor:	Yes, it is, but I just want to make sure I establish all your concerns before we discuss them in detail.

By separating out and exploring each concern the patient begins to see that there is some prospect that they can be tackled.

Breaking collusion

It is commonly alleged that relatives withhold the truth because they cannot face the pain of what is happening and wish to deny it. More commonly, however, it is an act of love. They cannot bear to cause anguish to their loved one. Approaching collusion from this perspective makes it possible to respect relatives' reasons and work positively with them. The first step is to acknowledge the collusion and then explore and validate the reasons for it.

Doctor:	You've told me that you don't feel Richard ought to know what is going on. Why do you feel that?
Mrs P:	I'm terrified that if he's told he'll simply fall apart. I wouldn't want that. I couldn't bear it.
Doctor:	Well, you know him best and you could be right. It could be that if he's told he will fall apart. Have you any other reasons why you feel he shouldn't be told?
Mrs P:	I think he'd just give up and turn his face to the wall.
Doctor:	Any other reasons?
Mrs P:	No.
Doctor:	So you have good reason for him not being told.
Mrs P:	Yes.

It is then important to establish the emotional cost of the collusion.

Doctor:	I now understand why you have kept the information from him, but what effect has this been having on you?
Mrs P:	It's been a terrible strain. I'm feeling extremely tense. I'm not sleeping as well as I should, I'm getting nightmares.
Doctor:	Would you like to tell me about your nightmares?
Mrs P:	He seems to be getting smaller and smaller, he seems to be wasting away.
Doctor:	That's, I suppose, what could happen, isn't it, given that he is dying?
Mrs P:	(In tears) Yes, it is and I'm very worried about it.
Doctor:	So it sounds as if you are finding it a strain!
Mrs P:	It is. It's a big strain. I worry that he will begin to guess. He's already commented that I seem quieter than usual.
Doctor:	Just how tense have you been?
Mrs P:	At times I feel at screaming point and I'm taking it out on the children. I feel bad about that, but I just can't see how I can tell him without his falling apart.
Doctor:	Are you experiencing any other problems because of not telling him?
Mrs P:	Yes, we're not talking together like we used to. I'd like to be extra loving to him, but if I am he'll guess. He says I'm backing off. But I can't explain to him why. It's horrible. Just when I want to be close to him a barrier is growing between us.
Doctor:	So, there are two good reasons for trying to consider whether there's some way round this, the strain on you and the effect on your relationship with your husband.
Mrs P:	Yes.
Doctor:	So, would you like me to suggest how we might be able to do something about it?
Mrs P:	But you're not going to tell him, are you?
Doctor:	No, what I'm going to discuss doesn't involve telling him. Would you like me to go into it?

Mrs P:	Yes I would.

You should now indicate that you would like to chat with her partner to check whether he has any idea of what is happening to him. You should reinforce that you have no intention of telling him and enter into a contract to this effect.

Doctor:	Let me emphasise that I have no intention of telling him. What I'd like to do is to chat to him to see what he's thinking about the present situation. It may be that he will reveal that he knows he has cancer. If that's the case, there will be no reason to maintain the pretence.
Mrs P:	But you're not going to tell him, are you?
Doctor:	No, I'm not. I will simply check whether he knows. If your hunch that he doesn't have any idea is correct, that's the end of the matter. I won't say anything.
Mrs P:	(Reluctantly) All right then.

Your next task is to establish her partner's level of awareness. You should ask an appropriate directive question that elicits his view of what is happening and then explore the cues he gives.

Doctor:	I wanted to have a chat to see how you feel things are going.
Mr P:	Not very well.
Doctor:	Not very well?
Mr P:	Isn't it obvious? I'm not having any more treatment. The hospital don't want to see me again but I'm still getting the pain. I'm losing weight and I haven't much energy. I'm in bed all the time now.
Doctor:	So, what are you making of this?
Mr P:	I think it's the end, isn't it?
Doctor:	Are there any other reasons why you're beginning to feel it's the end?
Mr P:	I've always known that what they've told me was a precancerous ulcer was a cancer. Now what's happening is confirming that I was right. I'm lying here just wondering why no one has levelled with me.

| Doctor: | It sounds as though you've known for some time what's happening. |
| Mr P: | Yes, I have, but I didn't want to upset my wife. She has enough on her plate with me being ill, and having to run around all the time. |

You should now confirm that he is right ("I'm afraid you are right") and then seek permission to convey his awareness to his wife, indicating that she knows the diagnosis. Then negotiate with the couple to see if they are prepared to talk with you to establish their concerns.

As you help the couple talk you may notice that the patient is angry with you. This usually indicates that he or she feels talking is a waste of time because it will not change the outcome of the disease. If you get this feeling, acknowledge it.

Doctor:	Would you like to say how this leaves you feeling?
Mr P:	What's the point? It's not going to be of much use.
Doctor:	It sounds as if you might be feeling that talking is no use because it won't make any difference to your situation.
Mr P:	That's right; it's not going to stop me dying, is it?
Doctor:	No, you're absolutely right. That's the one thing I can't do and I'm sorry about that. But it may help if we talk about how you're feeling and what you're worried about. It is quite likely there is something I can do to help you both. However, I will understand if you decide not to talk to me.
Mr P:	I suppose I've got nothing to lose by talking.

Breaking collusion is painful for the doctor who witnesses the love between a couple and the effects of imminent loss, but it is important to break it as soon as it becomes a problem. Otherwise important unfinished business will be left unresolved. Patients are then likely to be distressed and may become morbidly anxious and depressed. This mental suffering will lower the threshold at which they experience physical symptoms, such as pain and sickness, and cause problems with symptom relief. Failing to deal with important practical and emotional unfinished business also makes it difficult for relatives to resolve their grief. They are then at greater risk of major psychiatric morbidity, including the development of a generalised anxiety disorder or major depressive illness.

Challenging denial

Patients use denial when the truth is too painful to bear, so denial should not be challenged unless it is creating serious problems for patients or relatives. In challenging denial it is important to do it gently so that fragile defences ar not disrupted, but firmly enough so that any awareness can be explored and developed.

It is first worth asking patients to give an account of what has happened since the illness was first discovered and explore how they felt at each key point—for example, when they first developed the symptoms, saw a specialist, were investigated, and were told about the illness. They can then explain what they perceive is wrong, and thus may provide glimpses of doubt: "I'm certain it's an ulcer; at least, I'm pretty sure it is." By repeating "Pretty sure" you may prompt a patient to say, "Well, I suppose there could be some doubt." The cue "some doubt" can be explored next to see if the patient owns up to the possibility that the ulcer could be cancer. It is then important to interpret what is happening by saying "Part of you prefers to believe that it's an ulcer, but another part of you is willing to consider that it is more serious." Patients can then retreat to denial or develop their awareness further ("I've been trying to kid myself that it's an ulcer, but deep down I realise it's cancer").

If this strategy fails, look for and challenge any inconsistencies between patients' experiences and perceptions.

Doctor:	You say you were far bigger in this pregnancy than in your two previous ones. Did you consider why that might be?
Mrs J:	I thought it was just one of those things. I didn't think anything more about it.
Doctor:	Are you sure?
Mrs J:	Yes, I am sure it was a normal pregnancy. The reason I'm still feeling so weak is because I didn't take it too well.

This patient had developed ovarian cancer, which was so advanced that little treatment could be offered. She preferred to deny this and insisted that her symptoms represented normal sequelae of pregnancy.

If challenging inconsistencies fails to dent denial, check if there is "a window". Do this by asking "I can understand that you feel it is an infection. But is there any time, even for a moment, when you consider that it may not be so simple?" A patient may say "No", in which case you have to accept that the patient finds it too painful to look at what is happening. Alternatively, a patient may admit "Yes, there is. Sometimes I feel it could be something much more sinister." Exploring what patients mean by "sinister" may help them acknowledge that they have something much more serious than an ulcer. This then helps them shift from denial into relative or full awareness of their illness or prognosis.

Patients may oscillate between denial and awareness. Do not assume what stance they are going to take, but explore it each time by asking "How do you feel things are going?"

Conclusion

The best way to validate these guidelines is to try them out in your own practice. Either you will find they will work, and feel more confident about using them, or you will discover other strategies that work as well or better.

Acknowledgement

This chapter is based on work funded by the Cancer Research Campaign. Thank you to all those individuals who contributed ideas.

Index

Road Research Laboratory 60
road signs 60
role play 227
  briefing 228–9
  feedback 229
  problems in counselling 229–30
  rules 228
Royal College of General
    Practitioners 203
  Scientific Foundation Board 202
Royal College of Midwives 87
Royal College of Nursing 87
Royal College of Psychiatrists 68,
    72
Royal College of Surgeons 161
Royal Colleges 87
Royal Fine Art Commission 60
Royal Free Hospital 56, 58
Royal Postgraduate Medical School
    56, 64
Royal Waterloo Hospital for
    Children and Women 56

sabbatical from general practice
  awards, grants, scholarships 203
  exchange of practices 203
  family 201
  financial aspects 202–3
  locums abroad 203–4
  practice policy 201–2
  prolonged study leave scheme
    202–3
  reasons 200–1
  return to work 205
  spiritual refreshment 205
  useful contacts 206
St Bartholomew's Hospital 61
St Charles's Hospital 61
St George's, Hyde Park Corner 56,
    60
St Mary's Hospital 64
Save the Children Fund 191, 206
schizophrenia 67
scientific communications 153
service specification
  activity data 49
  aims and objectives 48
  definition 47–9
  description of service 48

facilities 48
format 49
monitoring 50
policies and codes of practice 49
quality 49–50
staffing 49
shorthand 31–2
sick doctors 66–8
  alcohol and drug dependence 67,
    68
  depression 69
  General Medical Council 72
  health education and medical
    profession 70
  helping 71–2
  problems in treatment 70–1
signposting of hospitals
  campuses 63–4
  carparks 57
  entrance 57
  Health signs system 55, 59–60
  lettering 59–64
  maintenance 59
  manufacture and cost 58
  maps and plans 57
  name boards 58
  other languages 63
  proclaiming name 56
  to the hospital 56
  wards, departments, lifts 58
Signs 55, 59–60
Sikhism 219–21
  imminent death 220
  signs 220
smoking
  employers 76, 78
  health hazards 77
  law and the workplace 77–8
  no-smoking policy 76–81
  passive 78
  ventilation systems 78
  voluntary codes 77
social workers 28, 29
Stillbirth and Neonatal Death
    Society 221–2
stillbirths 212, 214, 216, 219, 221
Stock Exchange 173, 174
stroke 77
suicide 67, 69